MW01673218

# Hypolipidemic Activity of Siddha Medicinal Plants

By

A Manoharan

## TABLE OF CONTENTS


| Chapter No. | Title | Page No. |
|---|---|---|
| 1 | INTRODUCTION | 1 |
| 2 | AIM AND OBJECTIVES | 5 |
| 3 | REVIEW OF LITERATURE | 7 |
| 4 | MATERIALS AND METHODS | 45 |
| 5 | RESULTS AND DISCUSSION | 81 |
| 6 | SUMMARY | 162 |
| 7 | CONCLUSION | 164 |

## DETAILED CONTENTS


| S.No | TITLE | | PAGE NO |
|---|---|---|---|
| 01 | **INTRODUCTION** | | 1 |
| 02 | **AIM AND OBJECTIVES** | | 5 |
| | 2.1 Aim | | 5 |
| | 2.2 Objectives | | 5 |
| 03 | **REVIEW LITERATURE** | | 7 |
| | 3.1 Studies on *Murraya koenigii* (L.) Spreng. (Rutaceaeae) | | 9 |
| | 3.2 Studies on *Gossypium herbaceum* L. (Malvaceae) | | 16 |
| | 3.3 Studies on *Curcuma longa* L. (Zingiberaceae) | | 19 |
| | 3.4 Studies on *Coscinium fenesrtratum* (Gaertn,) Colebr. (Menispermaceae) | | 24 |
| | 3.5 Studies on *Terminalia chebula* Retz. (Combretaceae) | | 27 |
| | 3.6 Studies on *Terminalia bellirica* (Gaertn.) Roxb. (Combretaceae) | | 30 |
| | 3.7 Studies on *Phyllanthus emblica* L. (Euphorbiaceae) | | 32 |
| | 3.8 Studies on *Salacia chinensis* L. (Celastraceae) | | 36 |
| | 3.9 List of Siddha Medicinal Plants with Hypolipidemic Activity | | 39 |
| 04 | **MATERIAL AND METHODS** | | 45 |
| | 4.1 | Study Material | 45 |
| | | 4.1a Composition of Karuvepillai Chooranam (KVC) | 45 |
| | | 4.1b Siddha Medicinal Plants of KVC | 46 |
| | 4.2 | Phytochemical and HPTLC Fingerprint Profile studies | 52 |
| | | 4.2a Phytochemical Analysis | 52 |

# TABLE OF CONTENTS


| Chapter No. | Title | Page No. |
|---|---|---|
| 1 | INTRODUCTION | 1 |
| 2 | AIM AND OBJECTIVES | 5 |
| 3 | REVIEW OF LITERATURE | 7 |
| 4 | MATERIALS AND METHODS | 45 |
| 5 | RESULTS AND DISCUSSION | 81 |
| 6 | SUMMARY | 162 |
| 7 | CONCLUSION | 164 |

DETAILED CONTENTS


| S.No | TITLE | | PAGE NO |
|---|---|---|---|
| 01 | INTRODUCTION | | 1 |
| 02 | AIM AND OBJECTIVES | | 5 |
| | 2.1 Aim | | 5 |
| | 2.2 Objectives | | 5 |
| 03 | REVIEW LITERATURE | | 7 |
| | 3.1 Studies on *Murraya koenigii* (L.) Spreng. (Rutaceaeae) | | 9 |
| | 3.2 Studies on *Gossypium herbaceum* L. (Malvaceae) | | 16 |
| | 3.3 Studies on *Curcuma longa* L. (Zingiberaceae) | | 19 |
| | 3.4 Studies on *Coscinium fenesrtratum* (Gaertn,) Colebr. (Menispermaceae) | | 24 |
| | 3.5 Studies on *Terminalia chebula* Retz. (Combretaceae) | | 27 |
| | 3.6 Studies on *Terminalia bellirica* (Gaertn.) Roxb. (Combretaceae) | | 30 |
| | 3.7 Studies on *Phyllanthus emblica* L. (Euphorbiaceae) | | 32 |
| | 3.8 Studies on *Salacia chinensis* L. (Celastraceae) | | 36 |
| | 3.9 List of Siddha Medicinal Plants with Hypolipidemic Activity | | 39 |
| 04 | MATERIAL AND METHODS | | 45 |
| | 4.1 | Study Material | 45 |
| | | 4.1a Composition of Karuvepillai Chooranam (KVC) | 45 |
| | | 4.1b Siddha Medicinal Plants of KVC | 46 |
| | 4.2 | Phytochemical and HPTLC Fingerprint Profile studies | 52 |
| | | 4.2a Phytochemical Analysis | 52 |

| | | | |
|---|---|---|---|
| | | **4.2b Determination of Moisture Content** | **55** |
| | | **4.2c Estimation of Extractive Values of Solvents** | **55** |
| | | **4.2d Determination of Ash Values** | **56** |
| | | **4.2e Biochemical Analysis** | **58** |
| | | **4.2f HPTLC Fingerprint Profile Method** | **58** |
| | **4.3** | **Antioxidant Activity Studies** | **59** |
| | | **4.3a ABTS Assay** | **60** |
| | | **4.3b DPPH Assay** | **60** |
| | | **4.3c Nitric Oxide Radical Assay** | **61** |
| | **4.4** | **Antimicrobial and Hypolipidemic activity Studies** | **62** |
| | | **4.4a *In vitro* Antibacterial Activity** | **62** |
| | | **4.4b *In vitro* Antifungal Activity** | **69** |
| | | **4.4c *In vivo* Hypolipidemic Activity** | **70** |
| | **4.5** | **Anti Diabetic Activity Studies of KVC** | **72** |
| | | **4.5a *In vitro* Antihyperglycemic Activity** | **72** |
| | | **4.5b *In vivo* Antihyperglycemic Activity** | **73** |
| | | **4.5c *In vivo* Antidiabetic Activity** | **77** |
| | **4.6** | **Cytotoxicity and Heavy Metal Analysis** | **77** |
| | | **4.6a *In vitro* Cytotoxity Study on L6 cell line** | **77** |
| | | **4.6b *In vitro* Toxicity Study on 3T3-L1 cell line** | **79** |
| | | **4.6c FTIR, ICP-OES and SEM Analyses** | **79** |
| | **4.7** | **Clinical Trial Study** | **80** |

| O5 | RESULTS AND DISCUSSION | | 81 |
|---|---|---|---|
| | 5.1 | Phytochemical and HPTLC Fingerprint Profile Studies | 81 |
| | | 5.1a Results of Phytochemical Studies | 81 |
| | | 5.1b Results of HPTLC Fingerprint Profile Studies | 91 |
| | 5.2 | Antioxidant Activity Studies | 103 |
| | 5.3 | Antimicrobial and Hypolipidemic Activity | 107 |
| | | 5.3a Results of Antibacterial Studies | 107 |
| | | 5.3b Results of Antifungal Studies | 111 |
| | | 5.3c Results of Hypolipidemic Activity Studies | 113 |
| | 5.4 | Antidiabetic Activity Studies of KVC | 124 |
| | 5.5 | Cytotoxicity and Heavy Metal Studies | 142 |
| | 5.6 | Clinical Trial Study | 154 |
| 06 | SUMMARY | | 162 |
| 07 | CONCLUSION | | 164 |

## ABBREVIATIONS

| | | |
|---|---|---|
| HPTLC | - | High Performance Thin Layer Chromatography |
| DPPH | - | 1,1-Diphenyl-2-picryl-hydrazyl |
| SOD | - | Super Oxide Dismutase |
| CAT | - | Catalase |
| FRAP | - | Ferric Reducing Antioxidant Potential |
| ABTS | - | 2, 2-azino-bis-3-ethylbenzothiazoline-6-sulfonic acid |
| MIC | - | Minimum Inhibition Concentration |
| ZIC | - | Zone of Inhibition Concentration |
| NO | - | Nitric Oxide |
| SEM | - | Structral Equation Modeling |
| MBC | - | Maximum Bactericidal Concentration |
| FTIR | - | Fourier Transform Infrared |
| CKD | - | Chronic Kidney Disease |
| CCl4 | - | Carbon Tetra Chloide |
| AST | - | Aspartate aminotransferase |
| ALT | - | Alanine aminotransferase |
| ICPOES | - | Inductively Coupled Plasma Optical Emission Spectrometry |
| LDL | - | Low Density Lipoprotein |
| HDL | - | High Density Lipoprotein |
| VLDL | - | Very Low Density Lipoprotein |
| KVC | - | Karivepillai Choornam |
| MPO | - | Renal myeloperoxidase |
| NCEP | - | National Cholesterol Eradication Program |
| HbA1C | - | Glycated haemoglobin |
| SAS | - | Statin Associated Symptoms |
| SAMS | - | Statin Associated Muscle Symptoms |
| HMG-CoA | - | Hydroxyl-methyl-glutaryl-coenzyme-A |
| CYP450 | - | Cytochrome P450 |
| DMBA | - | 7, 12-Dimethyl Benz(a) Anthracene |
| TBARS | - | ThiobarbituricAcid Reactive Substance |

# INTRODUCTION

# 01.INTRODUCTION

Siddha is one of the ancient systems of Indian medicine. It has been flourishing in South India along with Dravidian culture. It has been in practice for over 5000 years in the treatment of a wide range of human diseases including diabetes. According to Yugi Vaidhiya Chinthamani 800 (Mohan, 2006), and Sarabendhirar Vaidhiya Muraigal (Vasudeva Sasthri, 2005) and Sarabendhirar Vaidhiya Rathnavali (Krishnaswami, 2014), diabetes occurs due to alterations in the seven constituents of human body. It is physical constituents of the body "Udal Thatthukkal" which influence the three vital humours, vata, pitha and kapha (Shanmugavelu, 1988). Further, it is explained in the above Siddha literatures that among the ten significant complications of 'Madhumegha Avathikal' (diabetic complication), obesity is the major harbinger for diabetes.

According to the International Diabetic mellitus Federation (IDF), the number of individuals with diabetes in 2015 had crossed 415 million and by 2040 this will rise up to 642 million. According to the IDF, prevalence of diabetes in the world is about 285 million and is projected to rise to a level of 438 million in 2030 if no adequate prevention and control measures are undertaken. Further, it is estimated that by 2036, 844 million people will be affected with Diabetes mellitus. So, diabetes along with obesity is a major health concern of the world.

The ICMR India B Study (2011) also states that about 62.4 million people are diabetic and 77.2 million people in India are in pre-diabetic stage. Among which 4.8 million people are diabetic and 3.9 million people are pre-diabetic in Tamil Nadu. Among diabetes and its related complications, dyslipidaemia constitutes about 16%. Further, hyperlipidemia, hypertension and obesity give high risk for the progression of Cardio Vascular Diseases

(CVDs).The various researchers have concluded that 3 out of 4 (75%) diabetics suffer from dyslipidaemia.

As diabetes is a middle age related metabolic disorder, it is prevalent in 30-40% of people worldwide. It is an important disease that can be presented as hyperlipidemia and hypertriglyceridemia. Hyper-cholesterolemia and oxidative stress are the high risk factors for CVDs, Coronary Artery Heart Disease (CAHD), Peripheral Vascular Disease (PVD) and autonomic dysfunction. Studies by action to control Cardiovascular Risk in Diabetes (ACCORD) (2009), Fenofibrate Intervention and Event Lowering in Diabetes (FIELD) (2005), National Cholesterol Eradication Programme (NCEP), Adult Treatment Panel (ATP) III (2002) and IDF (2000) revealed that there was an increased ratio of morbidity and mortality among diabetic and dyslipidemic individuals.

In modern medicine, statin group of medicine is widely used to control hyperlipidemic conditions to inhibit HMG-CoA reductase enzymes, which play a major role by controlling the production of cholesterol in the liver. The excessive amount of cholesterol deposited (or) accumulated in coronary artery (Plaque formation) is more preponderance to CAHD. It is the main cause for Ischemic Heart Disease (IHD), Cerebro vascular disease (STROKE). The more oxidative stress and free radicals are involved in disturbing the normal metabolic process. So, the treatment of above conditions involved statin drug in modern medicine. The prolonged use of this drug will produce myopathy, increased blood creatine kinase (CK) level (Diana, 2018; Paul, 2016) and impairment of renal functions (Bianchi, 2003).

Diana (2018) and Paul (2016) had warned about HMG. CoA reductase inhibitors (Anti-hyperlipidemia) which produced very dangerous complications like statin associated symptoms (SAS), statin associated muscle symptoms (SAMS) and statin induced necrotizing auto immune myopathy (SINAM).

Bancha *et al.* (2015) did carry out a study on the effects of simvastatin on proteinuria and renal function in patients with chronic kidney disease (CKD). The study reported that simvastatin was possessing lipid lowering and anti-proteinuric benefits in moderate to advanced CKD cases. However, the atorvastin was highly contraindicated in CKD patients.

Michael (2017) and Emanuele (2009) had investigated on the pravastatin administration. The provastatin is found to be the most precipitating eczematous eruption mimicking psoriasis and atorvastatin (lipid lowering drug) results in the bad prognosis after its administration. Emanuele (2009) had further noticed that prolonged usage of atorvastatin has ended up in the induction of autoimmune disorders like SLE, Dermato myositis, Polymyositis, Lichen planus pemphigoids and DRESS syndrome.

It is found further that the consumption of statins causes liver cell injury and muscle toxicity. The recent research findings indicate that anti-diabetic Siddha medicinal plants are capable of decreasing blood sugar and lipids level in experimental models and are proved to be less toxic in animal models than that of synthetic chemical prepartions. So, the modern medicines, which have always been prescribed in the management of hyperlipidemia and diabetes, could be used with equally potential Siddha polyherbal formulations for effective control and management of diabetes mellitus and its related disorders.

Agasthiyar Gunavagadam (Madhavan, 2009), Gunapadam Mooligai Vaguppu (Murugesa Mudaliyar, 2006), Sarabendirar Vaidhiya Muraigal (Vasudeva Sasthri, 2005), Patharthaguna Chinthamani (Mohan, 2006) and Sarabedirar Vaidhiya Rathnavali (Krishnaswami, 2014) have discussed the therapeutic potentials of various Siddha medicinal plants. Interestingly, there are many Siddha medicinal plants and preparations used to combat hypolipidemia and diabetes. Howevever, Siddha physicians explain that Karivepillai choornam (KVC) has the twin benefits of hypolipidemic and hypoglycemic activities. The polyherbal formulation of KVC is found clinically effective in lowering the accumulation of lipids and in decreasing the glucose uptake, predominantly in the skeletal muscles, in a dose dependent manner.

Hence, the present research work has concentrated on both *in vitro* and *in vivo* studies on the hypolipidemic and hypoglycemic properties of KVC, in addition to analyzing its pharmacological actions, such as, antilipogenic activities in 3T3-$L_1$ mouse embryo fibroblast, and antioxidant activities by ABTS, DPPH and Nitric oxide radical assays. This research also includes phytochemical, pharmacoleptic and chromatographic analysis of KVC. The SMPs of KVC individually are reported to be significant in decreasing lipids and blood sugar levels. The clinical observation on prevalent usage of KVC in the management of hyperlipidemia has necessitated the research on its evaluation with regard to its antihyperlipedmic actions.

# AIM AND OBJECTIVES

# 02. AIM AND OBJECTIVES

## 2.1 Aim

Siddha medicinal plants play a vital role in the treatment of hyperlipidemia and diabetes. Several siddha medicines are polyherbal formulations. These medicines are known for their less or no side effects. The modern medicines, contrastingly, are found to have side effects. This drives the patients to take up the course of herbal medicines. Karivepillai chooranam (KVC) is a popular drug in the management of hyperlipidemia . It is sastirically prepared by combining the raw drugs obtained from eight (8) Siddha medicinal plants. The KVC has a beneficial role in lipid lowering and glucose uptake lowering actions. This warrants an intensive research to standardize the KVC drug by using modern investigations and prove its efficacy in the treatment of hyperlipidemia and diabetes.

## 2.2 Objectives

The following are the specific objectives of the present study:

1. To understand the phytochemical composition of the Siddha medicinal plants of Karivepillai Chooranam (KVC) and to document the HPTLC fingerprint profiles of KVC.
2. To examine the antioxidant activity of the KVC using the standard techniques, viz., ABTS, DPPH and Nitric Oxide radical assays.
3. To find out the antimicrobial activity of KVC against common human pathogens and to document the pharmacological analyses with regard to *in vitro* antiadipogenic activities of the polyherbal extracts of KVC and also record the results of Triglycerides estimation methods.

4. To confirm the antidiabetic activity of KVC by Glucose uptake assay in 3T3-$L_1$ and $L_6$ cell line studies.
5. To record the cytotoxic effect of KVC using 3T3-$L_1$ and $L_6$ cell line and to record the results of heavy metal analysis through FTIR, ICP-OES and SEM.
6. To conduct clinical trials by a prospective open labeled, non- randomized, single blind control study in order to validate the hypolipidemic Siddha drug KVC

# REVIEW OF LITERATURE

According to the concepts of Yugi Vaidhya Chinthamani 800 (Anbarasu, 1998) if diabetes is poorly controlled, it may lead to 10 important complications (Madhumegha Avathaigal), and obesity is the primary cause for the onset of diabetes and dyslipidaemia. Whereas, Agasthiyar 1200 has clearly mentioned that there exists a positive correlation between predisposing disease factors such as excessive consumption of fatty foods, obesity, and over-sexual desires, and the occurrence of diabetes mellitus.

A comprehensive literature review on the individual herbal constituents of KVC reveals the Hypoglycemic, Anti-oxidant, Hypolipidemic and Anti-microbial activities along with inhibitory effect of AGE ON AGE gene expression, and cardio protective actions help prevent and cure diabetes and hyperlipidemia (ADA 2015, Dhanalakshmi and Balamurugan 2014, Taskinen 1986, Sharma 2005).

### 3.1 Studies on *Murraya koenigii* (L.) Spreng. (Rutaceaeae)

The leaves contain Proteins-6.1; fat-1.0; Carbohydrate-16.0; Fibre-6.4; Mineral 2%; calcium-810mg; phosphorus-600 mg; iron-3.1 mg; carotene-12,600 i.u.; nicotinic acid-2.3mg; vitamin C-4 mg/100mg, oxalic acid and carbazole alkaloids. The leaves are a rich source of vitamin A, and calcium. Leaves contains 63.2% moisture, 1.15% total nitrogen, 18.92% total sugars, 13.06% ash, 1.35% acid insoluble ash, 1.82% alchohol soluble, 27.33% cold water (Prakash, V. 1974). Phytochemical screening revealed the presence of amino acid, proteins, triterpenoids, flavonoids, tannin and phenol (Dheeraj *et al.* 2014).

The free aminoacids present in the leaves include asparagine, glycine, serine, aspartic acid, glutamic acid, theonine, alanine, proline, tyrosine, tryptophan, gama aminobutyric acid, phenyl alanine, leucin and isoleucine, treaces of ornithine, lysine, arginine and histidine. The leaves also contain a crystalline glucoside, koenigin and resin. Curry leaf oil is deep yellow in colour with a strong spicy odour and pungent clove-like taste.

A large number of secondary metabolites such as alkaloids (murrayastine, murrayaline, carbazole), triterpenoid (cyclomahanimbine, tetrahydromahanmbine), coumarine (murrayone imperatoxin) and other phytocompounds (mahanimbicine, bicyclomahanimbicine, phebalosin) have also been reported in the leaves (Narasimhan *et al.* 1975 and Furukawa *et al.* 1986). The above bio active compounds possess antioxidant, L-Pancreatic lipase inhibitory effect, antiobesity, antihyperlipdemiea, kidney protective activity, antitumor, antimicrobial, analgesic, anti inflammatory, anti helmintic, anti diarroheal and hepato protective actions (Vandana *et al.* 2014 and Birariet *et al.* 2010).

Abishek *et al.* (2008) has worked on the Immuno Modulatory activity of Methanolic extract of M.koenigii. The result showed that the *M. koenigii* leaves have more humoral immune response and phagocytic activity by using Nitric Oxide assay. *In vivo* Cyclophosphamine induced Myelo Suppression in Albino mice (20-22gm) in 4 groups of six animals were used in this study. In test group of animals were feed with the extracts of 250 and 500 mg/kg, PO. For 16 days, control group was treated with cyclophosphamine (30 mg/kg, IP). At the end of study had shown the extract of *M.koenigii* which have significantly ameliorated WBC counts.

Baskaran *et al.* (2011) worked on the antimicrobial activity and phytochemical analysis of various leaf extracts of *Murraya koenigii*. This study comprised *Murraya koenigii* powder used (100gm/100ml) in hot water, ethanol, methanol, chloroform, ethyl acetate, acetone, petroleum ether, hexane extracts. The work concluded that better inhibition zone

(MIC) diameter of extracts against bacteria, *viz.*, *E. coli* (12.27±0 25, 10.07±0.12, 15.17±0.29, 16.20±0.20, 10.10±0.10, 6.0±0.0, 10.07±0.12, 10.20±0.20), *Staphylococcusaureus* (22.10±0.17, 15.07±0.16, 15.0±0.20, 12.13±0.23, 12.07±0.12, 10.10±0.10, . 28.17±0.29), were better *Klebsiella pneumonia* was highly sensitive in ethanolic extracts (12.17±0.15) compared to standard drug Ciproflaxacin (20.20±0.20). In this study, he showed *Micrococcus luteus*, *Pseudomonas aureginosa, Bacillus cereus* were also highly sensitive.

Nilima *et al.* (2011) worked on the methanol extract of 11 medicinal plant anlaysis of proximate composition and measurement of antioxidant activity. He analysed different parameters including phenolic contents ($R^2$=0.96). The polyphenolic constituents in the extracts were found more responsible for free radical scavenging capacity. Total phenolic and flavanoid contents had the best inhibition of DPPH, TEAC, ABTS and FRAP (Ferric reducing antioxidant powder).

Zhang (2010) and Thilahgarani Nagappan (2011) worked on the biological activity of Carbazole alkaloids and essential oil of *Murraya koenigii* against antibiotic resistant microbes and cancer cell line study, He performed antimicrobial activity of isolated carbazole alkaloids and essential oil tested on five strains of clinical human pathogens. The carbazole alkaloids exhibit the highest susceptibility with inhibition zone of 18.5±0.5 mm, 18.5±05 mm, 18.0±0.5 mm against *S. aureus, P. aureginosa* and *S. pneumoniae* respectively. The MIC and MBC in *K. pneumoniae*, the inhibition zone of 18.5±05±0.5 mm. The bioactive terpenes, positive inhibition to bacterial stains study showed range between 10.00 mm to 18.50 mm. The minimal value of inhibition (MIC) was 25.00 µg/ml against *P. aerugoinosa* and *K. pneumoniae* while 200.00 µg/ml was the MBC against *S. pneumoniae*.

The essential oil and mahanimbine was found to inhibit the proliferation of cancer cells through cell line study. Ic 50 values of 2.12 μg/ml,1.98 μg/ml and in the MCF-7, P388 and He-la cell lines respectively. Meanwhile essential oil of *M. koenigii* displays Ic 50 values of 6.00 μg/ml, 7.01 μg/ml, 2.83 μg/ml in the MCF-7, P-388 and He-la cell lines respectively. He found the cytotoxic effects of mahanine, mahanimbicine, mahanimbine and essential oil were determined by using cell viability by MTT assay.

Swati (2012) had conducted an *in vivo* study on the hepatoprotective potential of polyphenolic extract of *Murraya koengii* in $CCl_4$ induced adult male wistar rats (175±25 gms) in six groups, each group treated with 200, 400 and 600 mg/kg daily for 15 days. After 15 days, the animals were examined, He found significantly reduced ALT, AST, ALP, TP and Serum Bilirubin level which decerased from 165.8±10.70, 372.3±19.51, 357.0±6.46, 4.23±0.26 and 0.44±0.5 to 64.00±3.48, 127.5±13.03, 160.9±0.98, 6.56±0.36 and 0.10±0.04 respectively.

Dinesh Kumar (2010) and Vandana (2012) studies a reviewed the research on *Murraya koengii* plant. The review article showed that methanolic extract of *Murraya koengii* structures can contain six bioactive compounds, namely carbazole, mahamimbene, girinimbine, Iso maha minbine, murraya zolidine, and mahanine. *Murraya koenigii* stem showed the presence of mukeic acid (l-methoxy carbazole-3-caroxylic acid).

Swati (2012) carried out *in vivo* study on the Hepatoprotective potential of polyphenol extract of *Murriya koenigii* in $CCl_4$ induced Hepatotoxic adult male wister rats (175±25gm,n=6). End of the study showed high content of polyphenols in the ethnolic extract of *Murraya koenigii* leaves with a hepato protective, decreased oxidant machinery and scavenging free radicals.

Shiva Kumar (2013) has studied the antioxidant and biological activities of three morphotypes of *Murraya koenigii*. He has determined the methanolic extracts which showed good significant activity to scavenge ABTS and Hydroxyl Free radicals, Iron chelating ability and Total antioxidant capacity. The Iron (11) ions chelating activities of *Murraya koenigii*. $IC_{50}$ µg/ml was 337±5.6 µg/ml, 452±12.5 µg/ml, 126.8±01 µg/ml and 13±0.9 µg/ml. His studies showed extensively high antioxidant activity of *M.koenigii* by using molybdenum assay in three types. The antioxidant activities (AAE mg/g) are 621.2±3.88, 641±2.15 and 1268.8±1.71,which is The significant value at $p<0.05$.

Ali *et al.* (2014) has studied the bioactive compounds, pharmaceutical quality and anticancer activity of curry leaf. The results obtained from a preliminary analysis of Flavanoid compounds like Rutin, Quercetin, Epicatechin, Catechin, Naringin and Muricetin. The curry leaf has highest TF and TP contents with highest antioxidant activity as indicated by the FRAP and DPPH assays. He has studied methanolic extract of curry leaf extracts which exhibited a promising anticancer activity on MDA MB-231 human breast cancer cell line. The extract contained substantial amounts of effective flavanoid compounds. It has high potency of growth inhibition of breast cancer cell.

Priyanka *et al.* (2014) carried out *in vivo* evaluation of aqueous extract of *Murraya koenigii* in unilateral ischemia reperfusion injury in rats. 200mg/kg P.O of aqueous extract in *Murriya koenigii* was used (n=8 in 5 groups). Biochemical, urinary parameters were lowered after using *Murraya koenigii*. Aqueous extract of *Murriya koenigii* possessed both preventive and curative effects against RIR injury.

Javed *et al.* (2015) had found the antioxidant and hepatoprotective activity of methanolic extract of *M. koenigii* against $CCl_4$- induced hepatotoxicity in rats, the test group of animals were treated 50, 100 and 200 mg/kg once a day for 14 days. After 14 days, the results showed significant reduction in Hepatic Peroxidation (HO) increased tissue antioxidant enzyme and lipid peroxidation tissue biochemistry.

Mrinal Sanaye (2016) has determined the antioxitant effect and anticancer activity against human glioblastoma (U373MG) cell lines of *Murraya koengii*. He found ethanol and methanolic extract of *Murraya koenigii* had reduced the viability of U373MG cell line in human glioblastoma cells through apoptotic mode of action.

Kartik *et al.* (2017) carried out *in vivo* pilot studies in paracetamol induced hepato toxicity in male albino wister rats (10 to 12 wks, wt 180±20 gms) by using TBARS assay methods, Reduced GSH and catalase and SOP activity. He observed 100 to 200mg/kg/BD dose was significant in reducing in AST, ALT, ALP, TB levels. Hepato protective activity in paracetamol induced oxidative stress and hepatotoxicity in rat models, due to free radical scavenging activity of *Murraya koenigii* was evident.

John molly (2017) worked on the effect of curry leaves powder on the liver and renal function in women in hyperlipidemia by using $CCl_4$ induced rat model. A statistically significant decrease in liver, renal para meters was found ($P<0.001$, paired t test). SGOT and SGPT were down from (mean ±SE) 26.85 ±1.17 to 23.23±0.78,19.63±0.95, 18.80±0.88 and t value was 4.022, and 1.65 respectively. Renal parameters like urea, creatinine values are reduced in this study (mean ±SE, t test) 22.93±0.76, 20.75±67, 0.75±01, 0.70±0.01 and t test 3.898, and 2.105 repectively.

Kartik (2017) has worked on the the hepatoprotective and antioxidant activity studies and used *Murriya koengii* alcoholic extract in paracetamol induced hepatotoxicity in male albino rats 180±20 gm). Study TBARS assay, reduced GSH, Catalase, and SOD activities. So, *Murriya koenigii* has proved a good antioxidant and Hepato protective potential, serum liver enzymes was reduced in paracetamol induced hepatotoxicity in rats observed. The liver biopsy showed normal lobular architecture and normal hepatic cells.

Padma *et al.* (2017) has studied about the anti cancer activity of hydro-methonolic extract of *Murraya koenigii* and assed for cytotoxic activity in different human cell lines by performing MTT assay, growth inhibition by colony formation assay and the inhibition of the chymotrypsin (Ch-L) activity of the 26S proteasome. He did the *in vitro* assessment for *Murryaya koengii* which had a better control of human myeloid cancer cells (HL-60), Melanoma B6 and Adiramycin resistant P38 mouse leukemia cell lines.

Birrari (2010) studied about *Murraya koenigii* leaves extract (30mg/kg/day) that has significantly reduced body weight, plasma total cholesterol and triglycerides level. Balgia (2003) did study on antioxidant and free radical-scavenging activity of *Murraya koenigii*. Alcoholic extract in rat liver for antiperoxidative effects, treated group has gradually decreased TBARS from 400.09 to 125.66 nmol/100 mg protein in a dose dependent manner.

Muthulingam Nishan and Parthiban Subiramaniam (2015) reviewed the *Murraya koenigii* leaves that consist of 63.2% of moisture, protein was about 1.15% of nitrogen, carbohydrate 14.6%, total sugar, ash values are about 13.06%. The final study showed, the hexane, methanol and chloroform extracts of *Murraya koenigii* was highly sensitive to *Bascilius subtilis, S. aureus*, *Salmonella typhi* and fungal strain of *Aspergillus niger, Canadia albicans* and *Trichophyton rubrum*. In addition, water and methanolic extract of *M. koenjii* in alloxan, Streptozocin induced diabetic rats (50 to 100mg/kg/bw in 30 days). The end of study concluded the changes of lipids level and inhibitory effects of alpha amylase and alpha glucoidase levels.

Shanashmi and Cynthia (2017) have studied the *in vitro* antibacterial activity of *M. koenigii* in different extracts by using disc diffusion methods with compared standard antibiotics. The different extracts are Hot water, Ethanol, Chloroform, Methanol, Streptomycin, Pencilin, Kanamycin and Gentamycin. The MIC (mm) viz 19,12,14,11,7,2,6,8 respectively. They found that the Docking study in *Streptococcus* mutant organism was highly sensitive to *Murraya koenigii* leaf extract.

### *3.2* Studies on *Gossypium herbaceum* L. (Malvaceae)

The physiochemical characteristic of cotton seeds were loss on drying 5 %w/w, total ash content 4%w/w, acid insoluble ash 0.08%w/w, Water value extract 9%w/w, sulphated ash 5%w/w, PH value 4.5, (Ali Esmail and Ai-Snafi, 2018). The preliminary phytochemical analysis of cotton seed contained steroids, flavonoids, amino acids, protein, phenol and saponins (John and Devi 2015). Total flavonoid contents in the extract of seeds was found to be 410+0.74 mg quercetin. Mineral contents of seed included phosphorus 1.03-1.33, calcium 0.24-0.04, iron 0.02-0.03, potassium 0.94-1.07, magnesium 0.44-0.56 and aluminium 0.01-0.06, besides traces of copper, zinc, strontium and vitamin A,B,D and E.

Gossypol, gossypurpurin, gossypitrin, herbacitrin, bedaine, quercetin, carotenoids, vitamin E, phytosterols, peptones and phospholipids (Sharma 2005).

Arjit (2010) studied the antimicrobial activity of flavonoid from *in vitro* tissue culture and seeds of *Gossypium* species. He found that flavonoid of callus tissue showed the maximum antibacterial activity as compared to that seeds. *Gossypium herbaceum* was highly potent on *P.aureginosa, E.coli* and *C.albicans.* The results were compared with the zone of inhibition produced by commercially available standard antibiotics.

Sharma (2011) has worked on *in vitro* antioxidant activity of *Gossypium herbaceum.* It was confirmed with the by DPPH radical scavenging effect and reducing power assays. The DPPH assay showed more inhibitory concentration (Ic 50 μg/ml) in *G.herbaceum* ethanolic extract. It was compared with the standard drug ascorbic acid. The MIC value was 44.69 mm and 13.80 mm respectively. A Reducing power of hydro-alcoholic extract of *G.herbaceum* and Ascorbic acid 250 (μg/ml) concentration showed good reducing power 0.96 ±0.1327 and 1.38±0.0971 respectively.

Hari Kumar *et al.* (2012) had done a study on ethanolic extract of *Gossypium herbaceum* on Paracetamol induced liver damage in wister albino rats. All study groups were found safe upto the dose of 2000 mg/kg/bw. After completing the studies liver enzymes significantly fell in dose dependant manner. The histopathological examination showed mild hepatic degeneration with absence of necrosis in comparison with control group.

Velmurugan *et al.* (2013) has worked on anti hyperglycemic and hypolipidemic activity of *Gossypium herbaceum* leaves in Dexamethasone (steroid) induced Diabetic Swiss albino Mice (25-30gm) and wister rats (150-200gm). Each group treated with 200 mg/kg/bw ethanolic extract of *G.herbaceum* was used in 10 days. After 11$^{th}$ day, it was found that TG,TC, LDL, VLDL levels decreased and HDL level increased in diabetic model rats (Cardio-protective lipids) and peak values of serum sugar level significantly reduced in 77.53%, 71.82%, 69.48%, 73.42%, 72.65% , 70.49%. He found $LD_{50}$ was 200mg/kg/bw.

Alisnafi (2018) have studied *in vivo, in vitro* on hydro alcoholic extract of *Gossypium herbaceum* was reducing DPPH radical scavenging activity, DPPH-IC50 values were found 44.69 yg\ml and 13.80 yg\ml respectively, total flavonoid cotent in the extract was 410+0.74 mg and total phenolic content was 5.86+0.75 mg in dry material. Modification of phenolic hydroxyl groups on gossypol significantly decreases the chemical antioxydative ablitties of free radical scavenging activity, DNA damage prevention, and demonstrating that the hydroxyl groups were critical to antioxidation. Further he found the percentage of antioxidant activity (AA) of 26.62, 27.86, 31.09, 32.78 and 40.53 respectively. The DPPH value in ethanolic extract of seed was 53,80.34,85.83,91.60 and 92.81 (10,25,50,125 and 250yg/ml) respectively. The aqueous and ethanol extract was significantly (p-0.05) reduced sugar, cholesterol, triglycerides and urea in a dose dependent order (200-300mg/kg/bw) in rabbit models and histopathological examination confirmed the protective effect of *Gossypium herbaceum* against alloxan induced destruction of B-cells of pancreas in diabetic rabbits. He determined the aqueous extract of *Gossypium herbaceum* was safer side in nephron protective activity (200 and 250mg/kg/bw).

Gossypol possessed antiviral properties against enveloped viruses, including HIV-1,HSV-2, influenza and para influenza. Incubation of HTLV-III B strain of human immuno deficiency viruses.

Ayodeji Augustine Ola biyi *et al.* (2016) saught to determined about the inhibitory effect of *Gossypium herbaceum* aqueous extract in rat models. The inhibitory effect of α-amylase and α-glucoidase in rat pancreas in a dose depentant manner (0-88.8 mg/ml) and malanoldehyde (MDA), Homogenate was reduced (0.33-33mg/ml). This two things is considerable an antioxidant .

Monika Patel and Mishra (2018) studied the qualitative and quanitative analysis of phytochemistry by using Spectrometeric technique.The total phenolic and flavonoids contents was 0.145±0.00066mg/GAE/gm,0.473±0.0008mg/QE/gm respectively observed for this study. So, the phenolic compounds and flavonoids are most responsible to reduced oxidative stress and inhibited scavenging free radicals.

### 3.3 Studies on *Curcuma longa* L. (Zingiberaceae)

Turmeric powder has approximately 60–70% carbohydrates, 6–13% water, 6–8% protein, 5–10% fat, 3–7% dietary minerals, 3–7% essential oils, 2–7% dietary fiber, and 1–6% curcuminoids.

Phytochemical components of turmeric include diaryl heptanoids, which occur from numerous curcuminoids, such as curcumin, demethoxycurcumin and bisdemethoxycurcumin. Curcumin constitutes 3.14% (on average) of powdered turmeric, having variations in content among the species of *Curcuma longa*. Some 34 essential oils are present in turmeric, among which turmerone, germacrone, atlantone, and zingiberene are major constituents.

Suresh Babu and Srinivasan(1997) had carried out hypolipidemic action of curcumin, in STZ induced diabetic rats. When 0.5% curcumin was used in this study, it showed significant decrease in blood triglycerides (TGL) and elevated phospholipids level in diabetic rats models.

Srivastava *et al.* (1995) andSiddiqui*et al.* (2006) had worked in the field of curcumin studies. They found that curcumin inhibited platlet aggregation induced by platlet activating factior (PAF) and arachidonic acid with inhibitory effects on TXA2 and Ca2 mobilization. Curcumin was also found preventing the adhesion of platelets in brain macrovascular endothelial cells.

Vladimir Badmaev and Muhammed Majeed (2008) explained that curcuminoids derived from *Curcuma longa* has effective role in COX-2 inhibitors and inhibit the formation of inflammatory leukotrienes and toxic cytokines. In addition, that i*n vitro* curcuminoids were found to highly inhibit tumor growth, especially in colon, squamous cell, hepatocellular carcinomas and sarcoma cells. His clinical study included oral administration of 4.5gms/day for 1 to 4 weeks. At the end, the result showed *Curcuma longa* having effective role in the management and good control of autoimmune related skin disease and neurogenerative conditions.

Tehranipour and Jayasree (2009) carried out studies on neuroprotective effect of *Curcuma longa*. The alcoholic extract was used to study peripheral nerves degeneration after sciatic nerve compression in male wistar rats. The curcumin extracts of 100 mg/kg, IP, 3, 6, 9 times daily were administered in study groups (N=6). It is concluded that curcumin extract had the protective role in neuronal death resulting from sciatic nerve injury.

Annapurna *et al.* (2011) had determined the *in vivo* anti cancer activity of *Curcuma longa*. They found that 0.05% and 1% of ethanolic extract of turmeric had significantly inhibited the 7,12-DMBA induced mammary tumoriogenesis and reduced the incidence of cancer.

Suzyand Salama (2013), Koner (2009) found the hepatoprotective effects of ethanolic extract of *Curcuma longa* rhizome (CLRE) on thioacetamide induced liver cirrhosis in rats (180-250 gm). The study recorded the histopathology, immuno chemistry and liver biochemistry. The CLRE treated groups were compared with controls. The CLRE induced apoptosis inhibited hepatocytes proliferation and no effect was seen in hepatic C4P2E1 levels. The effect of CLRE on liver function tests in rats showed significantly reduced lipids in low dose CLRE (2g/kg/bw) and high dose (5g/kg/bw) with dose depending response.

Monaand Hanaa H. Ahamed (2013) carried out a study on the role of *Curcuma longa* methanolic extract on colon cancer-induced adult male Sprague-Dawley rat models. All the animals of 5 groups were treated orally with 437.5mg/kg/bw and 875mg/bw for four months. After four months, the histopathology of colon showed colon B-catenin and K-ras genes expression. Plasma TGF,Bcl-2 and serum CE4,CCSA-4 level were assayed by RT PCR and ELISA methods. The study showed that all the treated groups have significantly reduced COX 2, beta catenin levels and K rat gene markers.

Sai Krishna *et al.* (2013) did a study on the anti oxidant and free radical scavenging activity of curcumin determined by different *in vitro* and *in vivo* models, by using DPPH, Superoxide dismutase scavenging assays and nitric oxide radical scavenging assay. He found that for the DPPH assay, IC50 was 1.08±0.06 mg/ml, $H_2O_2$ IC50 was 10.08+2.01mg/ml, $NO_2$

IC50 was 37.50±1.54mg/ml. The Ferrric reducing antioxidant power assay(FRAP) was 1240±18.54 ym Fe(II)/g for Super oxide anion IC50 was 29.63±2.07μg/ml. The radicals in a dose dependent manner inhibited the erythrocyte membrane lipid peroxidation in the IC50 value of 12.02±1.03μg/ml.

Muhammed *et al.* (2016) has carried out patho-physiological studies on the reverse effect of *Curcuma longa* against the toxicity of Carbon tetra chloride on albino rats (230-280gm). Experimental animals were classified into five groups each containing 10 rats, each group treated with $CCl_4$ (1ml/kg/bw, IP) along with ethanolic extract of *Curcuma longa* (100mg/kg/bw, daily) for 30 days. After 30days there was a marked decrease in lipids and renal biochemistry.

Sarah (2016) studied the effect of oral administration of *Curcuma longa* extract on the alloxan induced hyperlipidaemia in diabetic rabbits and the results showed a reduced blood glucose level after the treatment.

Ekeanyanwu and Ediogu (2016) have done a comparative study on the lipid peroxidation and non-enzymatic antioxidant status in hypertension, diabetic and non-diabetic patients. They found in their study, a significant decrease in TBARS-MDA levels in the diabetic hypertensive patients compared with the normotensive patients and increase in TBARS-MDA level in hypertensive patients compared with the normotensive patients.

Alessandra *et al.* (2017) investigated the antioxidant dietry approach in treatment of fatty liver. They explained the importance and therapheutic value of antioxidant compounds (flavonoids and phenoids) in lipogenesis, lipid oxidation and peroxidation. Antioxidants play a vital role to control simple steatosis, nonalchoholic steatohepatitis (NASH), liver fibrosis, cirrhosis, non alchoholic fatty liver disease (NAFLD) and hepatocellular carcinoma. Further he explained Flavonoids have the most antioxidant activities in hydroxyl groups in the phenolic structure of flavonoids.They have the most beneficial antioxidative effects through several mechanisms. Indeed, they are able to target different pathways. Flavonoids are able to control de novo lipogenesis, inhibiting lipogenic proteins (ACC, SREBP-1, FAS and LXR) and increased lipolytic proteins (AMPK, PPARX and CPT-1). They are also effective scavengers of ROS and RNS (super oxide, hydrogen peroxide, hydroxyl radicals and peroxynitrite). Fucoxanthin and carotenoids are mediated through down regulation of various lipogenic enzyme activities and upregulation of fatty acid β-oxidation activity in fatty tissues and it will be stimulating. UCP-1 expression in white adipose tissue, UCP-1 is the proton gradient created by respiration and produce heat generation (thermogenesis).

Augustine Amalraj and Anitha pius *et al.* (2017) had carried out a comprehensive work in curcumonoids. They used 50, 250, 300 and 500 mg/kg/bw of curcumonoids was administered in rats to ascertain wide range of biological activities including antioxidant, anticancer and cardio-radio protective effects in various experimental models.

Panahi *and* Hosseini (2015) has carried a study about oxidative stress and inflammation activity in both gender with 500mg curcumin powder two times a day per oral administration. The changes of circulating concentration of protein and improved oxidative stress.

YUE (2015) worked on Anti angiogenic and Anti proliferative activities in Human colon endothelial cells and HMEC-1cells with administered 0.4-7.0μg/ml curcumonoids and

Ar tunrmerone. The Turmeric extract provided better anti angiogenic and anti proliferative actions observed.

Tanvir (2017) was studied about antioxidant properties in *Curcuma longa* by using DPPH and FRAP methods. In DPPH radical scavenging inhibitory action was IC50-1.08μg/ml and FRAP highest value was (4204.46±74.48μm, FE [II] per 100 gms.

Betull Kocaadam (2017) has reviewed about curcumin was suppressed Mitogen activity protein kinase in 3T3-L1 cell adipocytes. The macrophage infiltration, leptin receptor (06-R) in white adipose tissue, adiponectin also increased. The adiponectin is positive effect against obesity by decresing NF-Kb activity.

### 3.4 Studies on *Coscinium fenesrtratum* (Gaertn) Colebr. (Menispermaceae)

The Stem contains berberine, ceryl alcohol, hentricontane, sitosterol, palmatic acid, Olic acid and saponin (Datta and Mathur 1988).

Venukumar and Latha (2004) had recorded the effect of *Coscinium fenestratum* on CCl4 induced hepatotoxicity in male albino rats. The results showed that the liver enzymes decreased, and histopathologically the liver architecture recovered almost normaly barring slight deformity of hepatocytes and clearing of cytoplasm.

Nair *et al.* (2005) had studied the Antibacterial activity of methanol extract in *Coscinium fenestratum* by a using filter paper disc diffusion method. The results showed good zone of inhibition (mm) for *E.coli, Klebsiella pneumonia*, *Salmonella typhi* and *Staphylococcus aureus.* It was compared with standard control drug Streptomycin.

Shanmugam and Umadevi (2011) showed that the worked in ethanolic extract 300mg/kg/bw for 45 days in alloxan induced wistar albino rats showed anti- hyperlipidemic and anti glycemic activity.

Santhosh Goveas and Asha Abraham (2013) carried out a study of evaluation on Antioxidant activity of stem and leaf methanolic extracts of *Coscinium fenestratum* by DPPH and ABTS assays. DPPH scavenging activity ranging from 4.7±0.67% to 3.2±0.36%. The methanolic stem extract showed the highest scavenging activity at a concentration of 512µg/ml and a minimum at 2µg/ml. In the ABTS assay the maximum scavenging activity ranged from 9.3±0.56% to 69.3±1.76%. Leaf extracts and Ascorbic acid in ABTS radical scavenging ranged from 3.6±0.27% to 46.3±0.88%. The antimicrobial activity of aqueous and methanolic extracts of leaf and stem of *Coscinium fenestratum* was also assessed by *in vitro* agar disc diffusion method. The results of MIC and MBC zone of inhibition in *E.coli* (17±0.33mm), *S.aureus* (6.4±0.67mm) and *B.subtilis* (11±0.3mm) and 6.4±0.45mm) were recorded in the study.

Anitha *et al.* (2013) has determined the bioactivity guided isolation of various extracts of *Coscinium fenestratum* for antioxidant activity. The different successive extraction using various solvents like petroleum, ether, benzene, chloroform, ethanol and methanol. The ethanol and methanol extracts showed maximum absorbance 0.916 to 1.113 at 700nm. The above two extracts showed moderate to maximum antioxidant activity.

Divyasree Sandeep and Sakthivel Ramasamy (2014) carried out *in vivo* and *in vitro* study of Cytotoxic and Anti-Tumor Activities of *Coscinium fenestratum* extracts (25 to 100 mg/ml) in male Swiss albino mice. The extract had significant anti-proliferative activity in dose dependent manner. This was confirmed by the HeLa cells-MTT assays and mitochondrial apoptosis detection, and apoptotic cells DNA double staining methods.

Sreejit *et al.* (2014) worked on a new biosource for the multifunctional bio active molecule ecdysterone (20E), The presence of significant amount of ecdysterone in the stem was 0.22% and leaves 0.12%. Ecdysterone was confirmed by using HPLC, FT-IR and LC-MS.

Saranyapin (2015) and Thirupurasundari (2009) worked on cytotoxic effect of *cosicinium fenestratum* on human head and neck cancer cell line(HN31). They determined it using the water extract of cosicinium fenestratum compared to5-flurourocil (5FU) on human HN31 cell line,a metastatic squamous cell carcinoma of the pharynx. The result showed the decreased phosphorylation of p38 MAPK, pAkt and increased tumour suppressor protein p53.The IC50 on HN31 was 0.12/ml. The IC50 of 5-FU was 6.6mg/ml. So, CF extract has highly potent to reducing risk of cancer cells.

Kuntal *et al.* (2017) conducted the phytochemical screening for various secondary metabolites and antioxidant activity of various extracts in *Coscinum fenestratum.* The antioxidant activity was determined by DPPH and Hydrogen-peroxide scavenging activity, $IC_{50}$ values of methanol, aqueous, aqueous plus methanol extract of *Cossinum fenestratum* and Ascorbic acid (standard) were used in this study. DPPH Ic50µg/ml in scavenging assay was 52.43±0.024, 66.21±0.021, 42.38±0.012 and 4.87±0.030 respectively. Hydrogen peroxide ($H_2O_2$) scavenging activity in the above extract was found 54.22±0.014, 68.28±0.031, 46.80±0.011 and Standard Ascorbic acid was 9.18±0.020.

### 3.5 Studies on *Terminalia chebula* Retz. (Combretaceae)

Nadar TS and Pillai MM (1989) studied the effect of *Terminalia chebula* on the cysteamine induced duodenal ulcers in rats by increasing the beta glucuronidase activity in the Bruner's gland.

Badmaev and Nowakowski (2000) found the extract of *T.chebula* protecting the epithelial cells from the cyto toxic effects caused by Influenza A virus.

Jagetia *et al.* (2002) carried out the evaluation of the radioprotective effect of *Terminalia chebula*. The study was carried out 10Gy of γ radiation induced Swiss albino mice (30-36gms). The different dose of *T. chebula* were administered (0.5, 6.25, 10, 10.25, 12.5, 20, 25, 40, 50 and 80 mg/kg/bw) intraperitoneally. The peak effective tolerance of *Terminalia chebula* extract showed 240-280 mg/kg/bwt, the optimum protective dose of *T.chebula* was 1/28 with its $LD_{50}$ dose.

Ahirwar *et al.* (2003) found ethanol and ethyl acetate fractions of *Terminalia chebula* fruit extract used in atherogenic diet induced male adult albino rats (200-250gms). All three group of animals were treated with100mg/kg/bw. Group III (ethanolic extract and IMF) showed marked reduction in total cholesterol (mg/dl), TGL (mg/dl), total protein (g/dl) and increased HDL-C (mg/dl) viz 0.133±0.0191, 38.06±0.686, 3.76±0.0559 and 78.23±1.283 respectively.

Suchalathaand Shyamala Devi (2004) carried out the protective effect of *Terminalia chebula* against experimental myocardial injury induced by isoproterenol in adult male albino rats. 20 to 50mg/100g of the extracts were administered in all the study groups. The studies showed that flavonol, aglycone and phenolic contents prevented degenerative diseases including vasodilatory and inhibition of platelet aggregation action (cardio protective).

Farrukh Agil *et al.* (2006) worked out the antioxidant and free radical scavenging properties of *Terminalia chebula*, by ferric thiocyanate (FTC), thiobarbituric acid (TBA) and free radical scavenging assays. It was found that the methanolic extract of *T.chebula* reduced DPPH radicals and FTC the maximum absorbance was determined 6-7 days in 516 nm (absorbance). The Total phenolic contents estimated was 166.33±18.01mg.

Gandhipuram Periyasamy *et al.* (2008) found that the biochemical studies in STZ induced adult male albino rats treated with aqueous extract of *T.chebula* 200mg/kg/bwt for 30 days. The study showed markedly decreased plasma insulin level compared to the control drug glibenclamide. $HbA_1C$, plasma urea, creatinine also got significantly reduced. Further it was that observed *T.chebula* extract increased plasma insulin and C.peptide levels in diabetic rats. C.peptide has insulin-mimetic effects as it was the acting insulin receptors, it increases glucogen synthesis and aminoacid uptakes (Gurnberger 2004). The C.peptide promotes (insulin signaling) insulin action at low concentration and inhibits it at high level.

Kannan P and Ramadevi R (2009) carried out antibacterial activity of *Terminalia chebula* fruit extract in different bacterial strains by using disc diffusion method. T.chebula extract was highly sensitivity and MIC and ZIC in *Bacillus subtilis, S.aureus*, *E.coli,*

*Salmonella typhi, Pseudomonas and Klebsiella pneumonia* viz 11, 10, 12, 8,10, 9 (1mg/disc) respectively.

Rohini Ahuja *et al.*(2013) carried out a study in anticancer potential of *Terminalia chebula* fruits against enrich ascites carcinoma induced cancer in male adult swiss albino mice. The high dose of ETC (200mg/kg,orally) significantly reduced the tumor growth and ETC was also found to be cytotoxic in the *in vitro* parameters.

Bupesh and Manikandan (2016) worked on the *in vitro* assessment of Ag-NPs, by using cell proliferation assay, based on tetrazolium dye (MTT) method. The methanolic extract of *Terminalia chebula* was used in the silver nano particals biologically and in an ecofriendly way. The biosynthesized silver nano particals were explored against colon cancer cells and multi drug resistant (MDR) broadspectrum microorganisms. The nano particles were confirmed by using FTIR,XRD,SEM,TEM,analyzer. The anti cancer effect of Ag Np was higly potential at 10 microgram concentration.

Denna Priscilla and Jasmine (2016) worked on *in vitro* anti cancer activity of ethanolic extract of *Termalia chebula* by using GC MS analytical method. He found 64%MCF-7 cell line inhibition at the maximum dose of 400 to 500 mg, Approximately 50%, 60% and 64% decreased cell growth was evident after 24, 48 and 72 hours of inhibition respectively.

### 3.6 Studies on *Terminalia bellirica* (Gaertn.) Roxb. (Combretaceae)

Jagetia *et al.* (2002) had worked on the evaluation of radio protective effect of Triphala in the male Swiss albino mice (30 to 36gms). Test animals were injected with various doses, viz., 200mg to 1gm/1kg/bw for 14 days and was observed for acute $LD_{50.}$ The optimum radio-protective dose of 10mg/kg TE was found to be 1/28 of the $LD_{50}$ dose (280mg/kg/bw) which was well below the $LD_{50}$.

Elizabeth (2005) had done the work of antimicrobial activity of *Terminaliabellerica*. The methanolic extract in various microbial strains, methanol, crude extract (test drug) and Ampicillin (control drug) were used in this study. The study on MIC, MBC inhibition zone was nearer to control study. The methanolic extract of *T.bellerica* was highly sensitive to *S.aureus*, *S.pneumoniae, E.coli, P.aeruginosa* and *Canadia albicans*.

Evan Prince *et al.* (2013) and Gopi Sudhakar Kumar *et al.* (2010) have determined the protective properties of *Terminalia bellerica* against D-Galactosamine (D-GalN) induced hepato toxicity in male Swiss albino mice (25-30gms). All the animals were treated with 1000mg/kg/bwt I.P. The result showed reduction in SOD, catalyse, glutathione peroxidase, GR, GST levels. Glutathione levels increased in lipid peroxidation of D-GalN compared to the normal control group. He observed a reduction of peroxidation levels in D-GalN induced Swiss albino mice.

Aarti Saxena (2013) studied on antibacterial activity of chloroform and methanol extracts of Terminalia bellerica. Maximum zone of inhibition was observed for chloroform extract of *T.bellerica* used against Enterococcus faecalis (29mm) with MIC 10.4μg/ml and MLC 41.7μg/ml in gram positive bacteria, while gram negative bacteria showed maximum zone of inhibition in methanolic extract against *E.coli* (20mm) with MLC 83.3μg/ml.

Nithya Devi *et al.* (2014) has determined antimicrobial and phytochemical analysis of *Terminalia bellerica.* She used various extracts (aqueous, chloroform and petroleum). The result showed the presence of secondary metabolites like phenolics, alkaloids, flavanoids and tannins. The antimicrobial activity was evaluated using agar well difusion method against bacteria and fungi (*E.coli,P.Aeruginosa, Klebsiella species, Aspergillus niger and Aspergillus flavus*). The FTIR analysis has revealed the presence of phenols, alcohol, amines and carboxylic acid as functional group in Terminalia bellerica.

Sushma, *et al.* (2016) has done a research work in Triphala on a Murine model of Isoniazid and Rifampicin induced Wistar rats (150-200gms). The test drug Triphala was given orally at 250mg/kg and 500mg/kg/bwt oraly for 21 days. After 21 days she found drastic decrease in AST, ALT, ALP compared to hepatotoxic groups signified hepato protective effects of Triphala.

Furukawa *et al.* (2006) studied about the antioxidant activity of *Terminalia chebula* and *Terminalia bellerica* by using TBA, DPPH and FTC methods. It was found that the above plants contained phenols, flavonoids, saponins and tannins, which were responsible for their antioxidant activity.

Miori Tanka *et al.* (2016) has done extensive *in vitro* study on the antioxidant activity in *Terminalia bellerica* by using DPPH scavenging methods. In this method, IC50 was

7.2±1.2μg/ml. In addition, it significantly lowered mRNA expression, alpha tumour, alpha necrosis (**TNF**-α) and interlukine-1 beta cells. So, the above two pharmacological anti inflammatory actions are playing very important role to reduce coronary atherosclerotic plaque progression.

### 3.7 Studies on *Phyllanthus emblica* L. *(Emblica officinalis* Gaertn). (Euphorbiaceae)

The fruits are a good source of vitamin C, carotene, nicotinic acid, riboflavin, D-glucose, D-fructose, myoinositol and a pectin with D-galacturonic acid, D-arabinosyl, embicol, mucic, Indole acetic acid. Fuerther reports include the presence of growth inhibitors, phyllembic acid and phyllembin (fruits) and fatty acids (seed oil), leucodelphinidin, procyanidin, tannin(bark), ellagic acid,lupeol, oleanolic aldehyde(root), tannins, poly phenolic compounds, terchebin, corialgin, ellagic acid, alkaloids, phyllantidine, phyllantine (Tolonen,1990).

Sharma and Yelne (2005) had elaborately investigated on the physico chemical constituents of various medicinal plants including *Phyllanthus emblica* L.

Yokazawa (2002) has concluded that 10-40 mg/kg/bw of dried fruit powder of *Phyllanthus emblica* for 2 months reduces the hyperlipidemia and oxidative stress.

Raghu and Ravindra (2010) found antimicrobial activity and phytochemical study of various extracts from chloroform, diethyl ether and methanol and found *S.aureus* with MIC value of 0.261, 0.432, 0.512 and *Klebsiella pneumoniae* MIC was 0.342, 0.528, and 0.631 respectively for the three extracts. A standard control drug Streptomycin with MIC value of 0.0313 and 0.612 for the above two bacteria were carried out for comparison.

Mohammad Sheaib Akhtar *et al.* (2011) conducted an *in vitro* study in Type 2 diabetic patients. He used *E officinalis* powder. 1-3gms was administered to the patients for 8, 15 and 21 days, once a day before breakfast. The study observed that blood sugar and lipid (LDL) profile came down to the base line. For 0, 8, 15, 21 days, the blood sugar and lipid results were 286.5±23.2, 124.8±17.3, 111.0±11.4, 108.3±8.5 and LDL was 119.9±8.4, 124.1±8.0, 107.7±6.4, 58.7±2.4 respectively.

Krishnaveni and Mirunalini (2011) have studied *in vitro* in antitumour activity of aqueous fruit extract of *P. emblica* (50to 100mg/ml) in different human cancer cell lines (A549-Lung,HepG2-Liver,HeLa-cervical,MDA-MB-231-breast,SK-OV3-ovarin and SW620-colorectal) and IC50 value was 16.5mg/ml was most active in inhibiting *in vitro* cell proliferation.

Gupta Priya *et al.* (2012) evaluated the *in vitro* antimicrobial and antioxidant activity of methanolic extract of *Emblica officinalis*. The MIC Values recorded for *E.coli, S.aureus, K.pneumoniae, P.aeruginosa* and *Enterococcus* were 50, 50, 50, 25 and 50mg/ml respectively. DPPH and $H_2O_2$ were found to be 15μg/ml and for 32μg/ml and ascorbic acid, it was found to be 12μg/ml.

Lincy *et al.* (2013) carried out a comparative *in vitro* study of *Emblica officinalis* fruit in various extract (aqueous, ethanolic, acetone). ZIC of *S.aureus* and *E.coli* was recorded 0.3 μg, 1.0μg and 1.5 μg, 3.75μg respectively.

Alook De *et al.* (2013) had carried out an *in vivo* and *in vitro* study on *Emblica officinalis* extract induced autophagy which inhibited human ovarian cancer cell proliferation, angiogenesis, and growth of mouse Xenograft Tumors. The result showed significant increase in the expression of the autophagic proteins beclin1 and LC3B-I a, significant decrease angiogenic genes,1a (HIF-1a) OVCAR3 cells and endothelial cell antigen-CD31, positive blood vessels HIF-1a expression in mouse xenograft tumours.

Bhuvaneshwari *et al.* (2014) studied about hepatoprotective effect of *Emblica officinalis* and its silver nano particles against $CCl_4$ induced hepato toxicity in wistar albino rats. She found that $LD_{50}$ of Emblica officinalis was 300mg/kg and $CCl_4$ (2ml/kg/day) by using UV-VIS spectral analysis, FTIR, XRD and SEM analysis.

Amit kumar (2014) has studied about anticancer nanomedicine in triphala and *in vivo* study in aqueous extract of triphala (50mg to100mg/kg five times weekly), showed drastic reduction in Capan-2, BxPc-3, and Barc-95(mouse thymic lymphoma) human pancreatic cancer cells in a dose dependent manner.

Malliga Elangovan *et al.* (2015) worked on the antibacterial and antifungal activities of *Phyllanthus emblica* leaf extract by disc difusion method. The antibacterial activity of *P.emblica* extract concentration ranged from 1000µg to 62.5 and was compared with the standard drug Streptomycin (disc 10µg) and Amphotericin B (20µg). The study revealed that petroleum ether leaf extract of *P.emblica* has potential antibacterial and antifungal activity.

Waffa Ahamed (2016) and Hossain *et al.* (2012) had done a comparative study on the antibacterial activity of *Emblica officinalis.* It deals with the *in vitro* study about antibiotics against four pathogenic bacteria. The antibacterial activity of phenolic extract of *E.officinalis* against *S.aureus, Proteus sp, E.coli* and *Bacillus sp* at different cconcentrations were studied. The highest MIC zone was found against *S.aureus* which ranged from 16±0.57 to 33.3±0.3 at 10mg/ml concentrations while *E.coli* for the MIC, MBC was 10.6±1.2 to 22.6±1.2mm and for *Proteus sp* 8.2±0.1 to 20.3±0.57 at the same concentrations.

Vinayagasundram and Ramasamy Venkatraman (2016) has worked on authenticity pattern of commercialized *Emblica officinalis* using Thermal Decomposition and Elemental TGA-DTA studies. This study provided significant differences in the decomposition percentage of phytochemicals as 28.4% and 21.5% for genuine (AMGS) and market (AMMS) samples respectively.

Chinmoyee Deor *et al.* (2017) carried out a study on the hepatoprotective activity of *Emblica offiicinalis* in $CCl_4$ induced albino rats (E.O. extract 100mg/kg/bwt orally for 7 days). The clinical parameters came down to the base line at the end of the experiments.

Piyawan *et al.* (2018) studied the antiproliferative activities and phenolic acid content of water and ethanolic extracts of *Phyllanthus emblica* against HeLa, HT29, HCT116, MCF7 and Jurkat cells using an MTT assay and flow cytometric analysis of apoptosis induction and cell cycle arrest. Based on the study IC50 Value in ethanolic extract, water extract and both extract in Jurkat cells was 0.12-0.65 mg/ml,0.22-0.85 mg/ml and 0.12-0.85mg/ml respectively.

### 3.8 Studies on *Salacia chinensis* L. (Celastraceae)

Yoshikawa and Shimodel (2002) has worked on the polyphenolic constituents with lipase inhibitory and lipolytic activities in rat models to prove that polyphenols and effective hypolipidemic phytochemicals.

Dhanalakshmi R and Balamurugan (2014) has reviewed the hypolipidaemia and anti atherosclerotic activity of several medicinal plants including *Salacia reticulata.*

Choudhary and Vijaykanth (2005) determined the antimicrobial activity of root bark of *Salacia reticulata.* The control drug was Ciprofloxacin. Chloroform and methanolic extracts showed good results in *S. aureus*, *P. aeuroginosa* and *E.coli,* viz., MIC of 18; 20, 15; 22 and 16; 20, mm respectively.

Tomoko *et al.* (2011) worked on the effect of *Salacia reticulata* on obesity and metabolic disorders in TSOD mice. He observed the changes in body weight, visceral and subcutaneous fat. In addition, the Salacia extract had reduced NAFLD, NASH and decreased the blood pressure.

Mukesh and Patil (2012) did a work on hypolipidemic activity of *Salacia chinensis* root extracts in adult albino rats and 3T3-L1 adipocytes cell line study of wistar strain (150-200 gms). The study drug, aqueous extract of *Salacia reticulata* (500mg/kg/bw) and Standard control drug Simvastatin 10mg/kg PO were used. The study showed decreased serum lipid profiles especially in LDL, TGL and phospholipids.

Hebbani *et al.* (2004) found α-Glucoside and pancreatic inhibitory activity of Salacital. The result of Salacital plus has strong inhibition potential against α-glucuronidase ($IC_{50}$=30.43±6.66μg/ml), moderate inhibition potential against pancreatic lipase with an $IC_{50}$ value 1.32±1.2mg/dl.

Arjuna (2015) and Yoshinoand Kuoji (2009) has reviewed *in vitro* studies of *Salacia reticulata*. The clinical study exhibited significant reduction in $HbA_1C$ and plasma insulin level within 3-6 months.

Rana Gopal Singh *et al.* (2015) did a prospective *in vivo* study on the effects of *Salacia oblonga* on cardiovascular risk factors in chronic kidney disesase. The *Salacia reticulata* powder (1000mg twice a day, oral) treated patients showed significant reduction in CRP levels, lipids and blood sugar. So, *Salacia oblanga* has significant beneficl effects on multiple cardio vascular risk factors in both diabetic and non diabetic kidney disease (MRD) patients, particularly as a lipid lowering agent and as a modulator of endothelial dysfunction and inflammation.

Dhembare *et al.* (2017) carried out a study on antibacterial activity of *Salacia macrosperma* (Wight). The MIC and ZIC were recorded. *P.vulgaris* (6mm) from acetone extract followed by petroleum ether (8mm) from root extract with high ZIC (15mm) were observed.

Godam *et al.* (2018) have studied the effect of ethanolic extract of *Salacia reticulata* on mercury chloride ($HgCl_2$) induced cellular damage of adult male mice. All the animals were observed by learning and memory test (Y-maze alternation test). End of the study showed, *S.reticulata* has potentiating effects in ameliorating the harmful effects of mercury chloride on the neural cells and cellular architecture. Godam *et al.* (2018) have studied the antidegenerative and neurobehavioral effects of ethanolic root extract of *Salacia reticulata* on mercury chloride induced cellular damage in the hippo campus of adult male mice.

Tsutomin Shimada *et al.* (2014) has done a research on a 12 week old TSOD mice in immature 3T3-L1 adipocytes. The mRNA expression of lipogenesis factor and adiponectin upgraded and enhanced the expression of total AMPK in mature adipocytes.

Ramakrishna *et al.* (2018) has evaluated the antidiabetic properties by using elicitor application and he found eight new compouds from abiotic elicitor. Further they described the eight compounds. The Cyclotrisiloxane and Hexamethyl were the main active molecules to control the free radicals and antagonistic effects.

## 3.9 List of Siddha Medicinal Plants with Hypolipidemic Activity

Various Siddha medicinal plants with anti daiabetic and anti lipogenic activities evidenced through clinical practice have been recorded in the literatures of Siddha system of medicine . A compilation of familiar Siddha medicinal plants with hypolipidemic activity is presented in the Table 1.

**Table 1** Summary of Siddha medicinal plants with reported hypolipidemic activity by Siddha literatures. *Ref No: 1 Gunapada Mooligai, 2 Theran Yamaha Venba, 3 Theran Kappiyam, 4 Theran gunabadam, 5 Agasthiyar Gunavagadam, 6 Pathartha Gunavagadam , 7 Pathartha Guna Chinthamani, and 8 Theran Maha Karisal(Thiyagarajan, 1997).

| S.No | Tamil Name | Botanical Name | Family | Part Used | Important Alkaloids | *Ref No |
|---|---|---|---|---|---|---|
| 1. | MangaiInji | *Curcuma amada* Roxb. | Zingiberaceae | Rhizome | β,d, Curcumene,<br>d-Pinene, d Camphor,<br>β - d - curcumene, Phytosterol | 5 |
| 2. | NilaPoosani | *Ipomea masritiana* Jacq. | Convolulaceae | Root | Puerarin, Tuberostan, Cardiac glycoside | 2 |
| 3. | Seenthil | *Tinospora cordifolia* (Wild.)Hk. f. & Th. | Menispermaceae | Stem | Tino Cardifolin, Tinosporidine, Tinosporaside, Cleodane | 5 |
| 4. | Kalarchikai | *Caesalpinia bonduc* (L.) | Caesalpiniaceae | Fruit, leaf | α, β and δ Caesalpins, Pentacyclic, | 4,5 |

|  |  |  |  |  |  |  |
|---|---|---|---|---|---|---|
|  |  | Roxb. |  |  | Tri Terpenoid (+) Ononitd, Cephanone |  |
| 5. | Vengayam | *Allium cepa* L. | Alliaceae | Bulb | Quercetin, Cycloallin, Phenolic Acid | 5 |
| 6. | Vellai- Poondu | *Allium sativum* L. | Alliaceae | Bulb | Ajuene, Y-glutamyl peptides, F-gitonin, degalactotigonin | 3,5 |
| 7. | Shengam | *Capparis decidua* (Forsk.) Edgew. | Capparaceae | Bark, fruit | Capparilline, N-triacontanol, Capparisinine | 1,2,5, |
| 8. | LavangaPattai | *Cinna momumverum.*J.S.Presl | Lauraceae | Leaf | Eugenol, Lianlool, Benzaldehyde, Benzyl Cinnamaldehyde, Pinene, Cymene | 1 |
| 9 | Kungiliyam | *Commiphora mukul* (Enzler) | Burseraceae | Resin | Resins, Z-Guggulusterone, EGuggulusterone, Guggulsterol I-V | 1,5 |
| 10. | Vellarugu | *Enicostema axillare* (Lam.) Raynal. | Gentinaceae | Whole plant | Swertiamarin, Gentiamine, Swertisin5-0, Glycosyleswertisin, 12Myristic acid | 1,5 |
| 11. | KodamPuli | *Garcinia combogia* Desr. | Clusiaceae | Fruit | Hydroxycitric Acid, Tartaric acid | 1 |
| 12. | Kostum/kottam | *Costus speciosus* | Costaceae | Root | Costunolide, dehydrocostus, Lactone | 1,4,5 |
| 13. | Vendhayam | *Trigonella foenum & T. gracenum* (Linn.) | Papilionaceae | Seed | GraecunninsA-G, Trigofenosides, Gitogenin, C-trigonelline, Quercetin | 1,3,5 |
| 14. | Kovai | *Coccinia grandis* (L.) Voigt. | Curcurbitaceae | Leaves, fruit, root | Lupeol, cucurbitacin, β-sitosterol, β-carotene, Linoleic, Oleic acids | 5,6,7 |

| | | | | | | |
|---|---|---|---|---|---|---|
| 15. | ChottuKathalai | *Aloe vera* (L.) Burm. f. | Liliaceae | Leaves | Aloesone, aloesin, barbuloin, glycoside, β-barbaloin, iso-emodin | 5,6,7 |
| 16. | Perarathai | *Alpinia galangal* Sw. | Zingiberacae | Rhizome | Methyl cinnamate, cineol, caryophyllenol | 4,5 |
| 17. | Vaivilangam | *Embeli aribes* Burm. f. | Myrsinaceae | Fruit, seed | Embelin, Quercitol, vilangin, Christembine | 2,6 |
| 18. | NallaThulasi | *Ocimum tenuiflorum* L. | Lamiaceae | Leaves | Stigmasterol, Volatile oil, Caryophyllene | 3,4 |
| 19. | Narivengai | *Ougenia oojeinensis* (Roxb.) Hochr. | Papilionaceae | Bark | Lupeol , Betulin, Homoferreirin, Ougenin | 4 |
| 20. | Agati | *Sesbania grandiflora* (L.) Poir. | Papilionaceae | Leaves, flower | Oleanolic acid, Galactose, Glucuronic acid, Cyanidin 3 – glucoside | 5,8 |
| 21. | Vengai | *Pterocarpus marsupium* Roxb. | Papilionaceae | Leaves, stem | Liquiritigenin, garbauzol, Glucosides, Aurane | 1,2 |
| 22. | Naayuruvi | *Achyranthes aspera,* Linn. | Amaranthaceae | Leaves | Oleanolic acid, ecdysone, ecdysterone, achyranthine | 4,5 |
| 23. | AlisiVirai | *Linum usitatissimum* Linn. | Linaceae | Seed | Phenylpropanoid, glucoside, Linnsitamarin, linseed oil | 1 |
| 24. | Adhividaiyam | *Aconitum heterophyllum* Wall-ex Royle | Rananculaceae | Leaves, stem | 3-0-β-D- glucopyranoside 7-0-β-D-glucopyranosyl -(1→3), quercetin 3-0-β-D-(1→3) glucopyrnoside -7- 0- (6E-Cafferyl) β-D (1→3) | 1,5 |

| | | | | | | |
|---|---|---|---|---|---|---|
| 25. | Itti | *Dalbergia latifolia* Roxb. | Papilionaceae | Bark | Methyl dalbergin , rotenoid, dalbinol | 1,5 |
| 26. | Pulichhai | *Hibiscus cannabinus* Linn. | Malvaceae | Leaves, seed | Isoquercitrin, Cannabiscitrin, myricetin, phosphonolipids | 1,5,6 |
| 27. | Karisalai | *Eclipta prostrata* (L.) | Asteraceae | Whole plant | Terthienyl aldehyde ecliptal, Nicotine, Triterpenoid | 1,5 |
| 28. | KaatuMurangai | *Moringa oleifera* (Lam.) | Moringaceae | Leaves, flower | Quercetin,3-Rhamnoglucoside, Kaempferol | 3,5 |
| 29. | NattuRuthratcha m | *Elaeocarpus sphaericus* L. | Elaeocarpaceae | Fruit, leaf | (-)-Isoleae, Carpilline, Rudrakine, Fixed oil | 1,5 |
| 30. | Pavakai | *Momordica charantia* (Linn.) | Cucurbitaceae | Fruit, leaf | Acylglucosyl sterols | 3,5 |
| 31. | Jatamanjil | *Nardosta chysjatamansi* (D.Don) Dc. | Valerianaceae | Rhizome | Jatamansone, Sequitepene, Angelicin, Jatamansin | 1,5 |
| 32. | Kothamalli | *Coriandrum sativum* (Linn.) | Apiaceae | Leaves, seed | Furoisocumarins, Coriandrin, Coriandrol, D.Mannitol | 5 |
| 33. | Naval | *Syzygium cumini* (L.) Skeels | Myrtaceae | Fruits, seed | Myrecetin-3-0 glucoside, Robinoside, Isoquercetin, Anthocyanins | 5,3,4 |
| 34. | Karuncheeraga m | *Nigella sativa* Linn. | Ranunculaceae | Seed | Dithymoquinone, Nigilline, Aarmacenine, | 5 |

| | | | | | | |
|---|---|---|---|---|---|---|
| | | | | | Trans anetholic | |
| 35. | Shenkottai | *Semecarpus anacardium* Linn. f. | Anacardiaceae | Fruit | Bhilwanol, Binaringenin, Semecarpetin, Galluflavanone | 3,5 |
| 36. | Vasambu | *Acorus calamus* Linn. | Araceae | Rhizome | Callaminone, Isocalamendiol, Asarone-3, β-asarone | 4,5 |
| 37. | Arugampulla | *Cynodon dactylon* (L.) Pers. | Poaceae | Whole plant | Apigenin, Luceolin, Orientin, Vitexin | 4,5 |
| 38. | Peerkankai | *Luffa cylindrica* (L.)M.Roem. | Cucurbitaceae | Tender fruits | SaponinsLucyosides A, H, Cucurbitacin B | 1,5 |
| 39. | Mandari | *Bauhinia purpureae* Linn. | Caesalpiniaceae | Flower | Tannin, Isoquercitrin, Quercitrin, Chalcone glycoside | 1,5,6 |
| 40. | Sarkarai Vembu | *Scorparia dulcis* Linn. | Scrophulariaceae | Scrophular iaceae | ScrophulariaceaeScoparic acid, Scopadulciol, Amellin, Root,.Mannitol | 1,5 |
| 41. | PulichaiKeerai | *Hibiscus sabdariffa* Linn. | Malvaceae | Leaves, seed | Citric acid, d - malic, Hibiscus acid, Gossypetin, Sabdaritrin | 5,6,7 |
| 42. | Nerunjil | *Tribulu sterrestris* L. | Zygophyllaceae | Whole plant | Diosgenin, giogenin, Chlorogenin, Tribuloside | 1,6 |
| 43. | Kollu | *Macrotyloma uniflorum* (Lam.) Verdc. | Fabaceae | Seeds | Dulichin A and B | 3,5 |
| 44. | Musumusukkai | *Muklamadera spatana* (Linn.) M. Roem. | Curcurbitaceae | Leaves, Root | Umbelliferone, Xanthotoxol, Isopimpinellin, Scopoletin | 5,7 |

| | | | | | | |
|---|---|---|---|---|---|---|
| 45. | Vilvam | *Aegle marmelos* (Linn.) Corr. | Rutaceae | Whole plant | Psoralen, Xantho toxin, Scopoletin, Siummianine | 2,5 |
| 46. | Chenthatti | *Tragia involucrata* Linn. | Euphorbiaceae | Root | Ethylbenzene, Limonene, TragiaSapomine, | 1,5 |
| 47. | Sirukurin Jan | *Gymnem asylvestre* (Retz.) R.Br.ex. Schult. | Asclepiadaceae | Leaves | Gymnemasins A. D., Gymnimagenine, Gymnemic acid, Gypenosides II, Nonacosane | 1 |
| 48. | NathaiChuri | *Spermacoce hispida* Linn. | Rubiaceae | Seed | Isorhamnetin | 1,8 |
| 49. | Illanthai | *Ziziphus mauritiana* Lam. | Rhamnaceae | Leaves | Jujuboside A, B., Jubanine A, B., Rutin, Ziziphin, Stephanine, Vit C | 5,6,7 |

# MATERIALS AND METHODS

# 4. MATERIALS AND METHODS

## 4.1 Study Materials

Karivepillai chooranam (KVC), which is a poly herbal formulation, consists of eight (8) Siddha Medicinal Plants (SMPs). These 8 SMPs and their useful parts which form the basis of poly herbal formulation of KVC (Table 1) were used in the preparation of KVC and the freshly prepared KVC was used as the study material for this study aimed at finding out the hypolipidemic activity.

### 4.1a Composition of Karivepillai Chooranam (KVC)

The details of the SMPs which form the ingredients of KVC preparation as per Sarabenthira Vaidhya Ratinavali Part II (Krishnaswami, 2014) are presented in Table 1. The raw drugs were purified, pounded and made into a fine powder. The powder was sieved using a fine cloth (Fig 2) before storing it in an air tight container for future use in the experimental analyses.

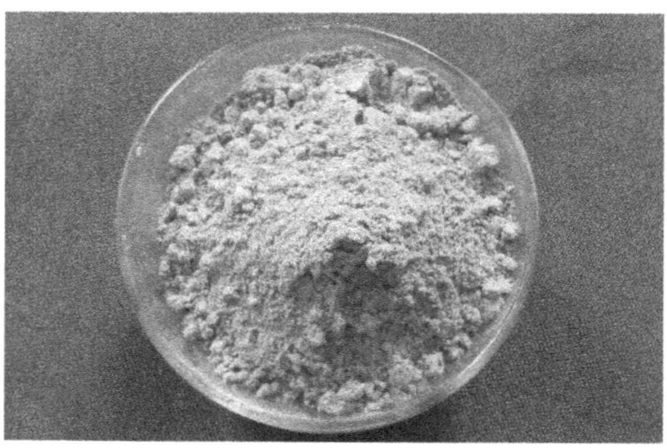

**Fig 2** The freshly prepared Karivepillai chooranam (KVC) used in the experiments

**4.1b Siddha Medicinal Plants of KVC**

The plant materials were collected from the Kalakkad Forests of Tirunelveli District, Marunthuvazh Malai of Kanyakumari District in Tamil Nadu and Santhigiri of Trivananthapuram of Kerala State. The vouchers of the 8 plants were prepared and identified using pertinent Floras (Gamble, 1957; Henry *et al.*, 1989; Matthew, 1983; Yoganarasimhan, 2000). The medicinally useful parts of the 8 SMPs collected at the time of KVC drug preparation are individually described below.

(i) *Murraya koenigii* (L.) Spreng. (Rutaceaeae)

The plant is an aromatic shrub or a small tree with dark brown or black bark. Its leaves are imparipinnate with the leaflets rhomboid, ovate or lanceolate, and gland-dotted (Fig 3). The flowers are white, in terminal, corymbose cymes. The fruits are berry, subglobose, and purplish-black. It is found in most districts and often cultivated (Matthew, 1991).

(a) (b)

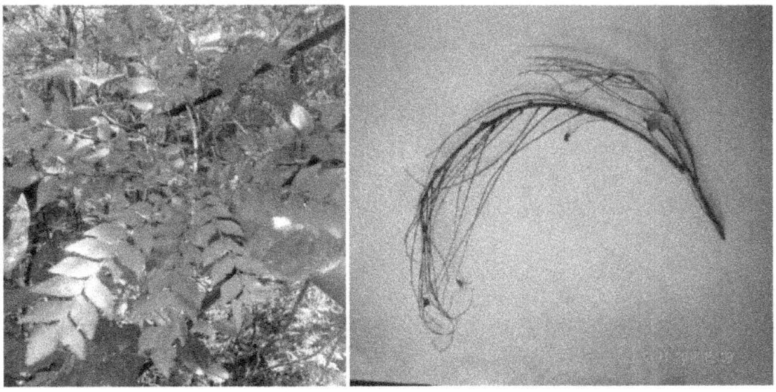

**Fig 3** (a) The Vegetative Twig and (b) Rachis Of *Murraya koenigii* Used In KVC

The leaves, root and bark of *Murraya koenigii* are tonic, stomachic and carminative. The leaves are also used in diarrhoea and dysentery and for checking vomiting. Root juice is taken for relief from renal pains (Yoganarasimhan, 2000).

(ii) *Gossypium herbaceum* L. (Malvaceae)

Habit-wise, the plant is a small shrub with stiff stems. Its leaves are 3 to 7-lobed. Flowers yellow with purplish centre, rarely white. The fruit is a capsule, globose and beaked. The seeds are ovoid and brown (Fig 4). It is distributed in all the districts of Tamil Nadu and commercially cultivated in the tropics (Matthew, 1991).

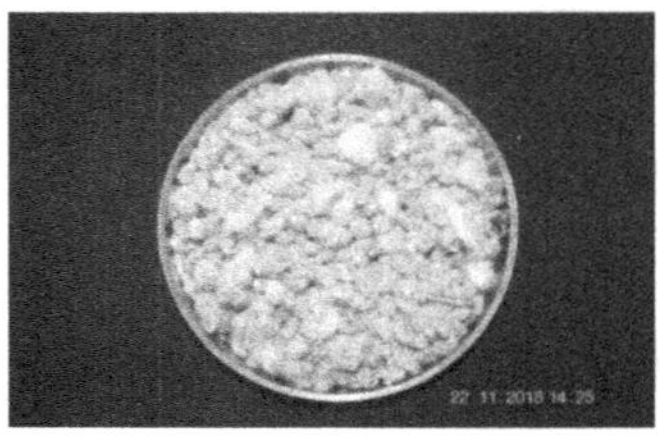

**Fig 4** The Seeds Of *Gossypium herbaceum* Used In KVC

In Siddha system of medicine, the leaf, flower, cotton, seed, stem bark and root bark of *Gossypium herbaceum* (parutti) are used in treating leucorrhoea, ulcers, swellings, fevers, dysentery, piles and cut wounds, besides their use as aphrodisiac (Yoganarasimhan, 2000).

(iii) *Curcuma longa L.* (Zingiberaceae)

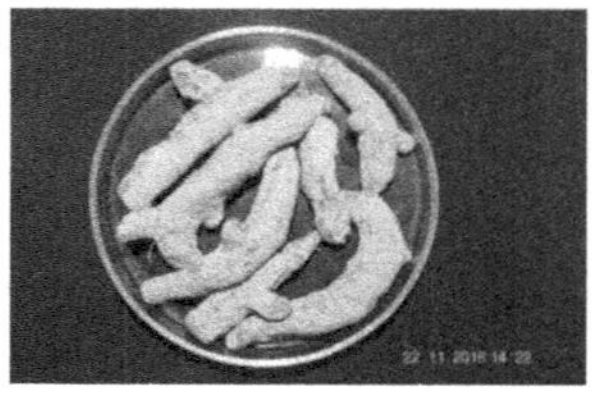

**Fig 5** The Rhizomes Of *Curcuma longa* Used In KVC

They are herbs with modified stems called rhizomes. The cylindrical, branched and tuberous rhizomes (Fig 5) bear large leaves in tufts. The flowers are in spikes with pinkish bracts. They are cultivated in most of the districts of India and in tropics (Mathew 1991). Rhizome is the source of turmeric used as a stimulant, tonic, stomachic and depurative.

In Siddha, the rhizomes are used to cure vomiting, headache, sinusitis, coryza, leucoderma, convusion, swellings, ulcers, pox skin diseases, fever, jaundice and eye diseases. (Yoganarasimhan, 2000).

(iv) *Coscinium fenestratum*

It is a large woody climber with bright tonic yellow sap. Its leaves are subpeltate. It is distributed in Nilgiri, Tamil Nadu entire south India and Sri Lanka. The stem (Fig 6) is used in digestive disorders, fever, piles, diseases of pittam and contusion (Yoganarasimhan, 2000).

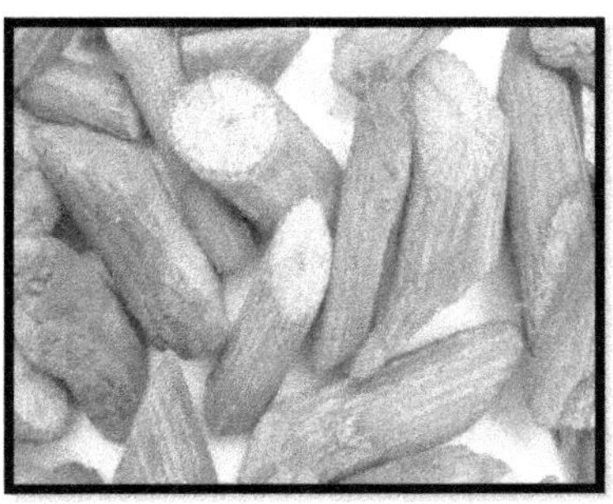

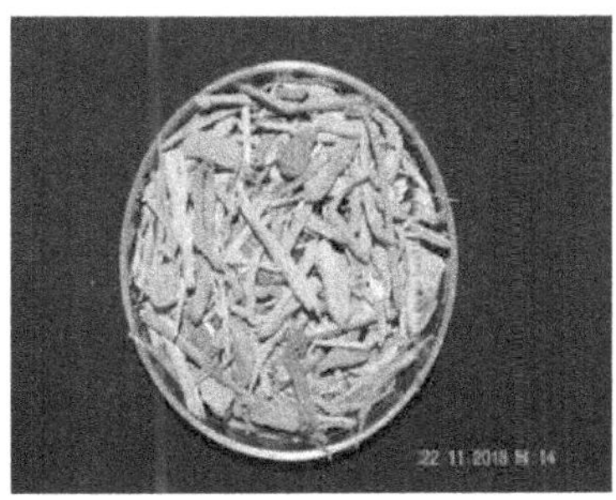

**Fig 6** The Stems Of *Coscinium fenestratum*: (a) Before Drying And (b) After Drying

The cut stems of *Coscinium fenestratum* after shade drying are used in the preparation of KVC.

(v) *Terminalia chebula* Retz. (Combretaceae)

The plants are large deciduous trees with dark-brown, cracked bark, exfoliating in woody scales. The leaves are elliptic-obobate, densely woolly beneath, with 2 basal glands. The flowers are yellowish-white and in axillary spikes. The fruits are drupe, obovoid and ornage-brown (Fig 7). They are found growing in almost all districts of Tamil Nadu and in India, Sri Lanka, Nepal and Burma (Matthew, 1991).

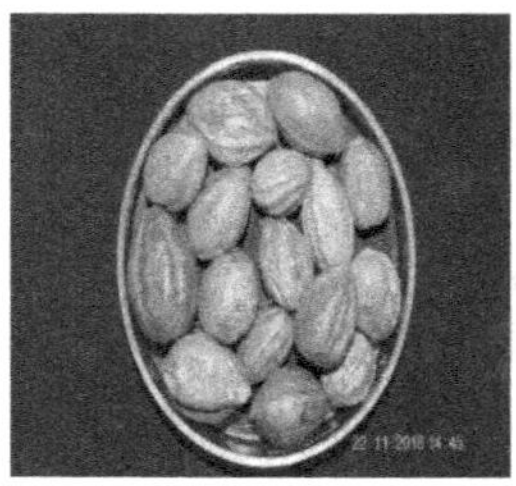

**Fig 7** The Dried Fruits Of *Terminalia chebula* Used In KVC

According to Siddha medicine, the fruits help cure Jaundice, poisoning, obesity, polyuria, anorexia, cardiac diseases, haemorrhage, eye diseases, cough, dyspnoea, ascites, urinary disorders and carcinoma, besides being used as a rejuvenator (Yoganarasimhan, 2000).

(v) *Terminalia bellirica* (Gaertn.) Roxb. (Combretaceae)

The individuals of *Terminalia bellirica* are large buttressed deciduous trees, whose leaves are broadly ovate without glands. The flowers are creamy-white born in axillary spikes. The shape of fruit is ovoid, slightly 5-ridged, brown and pubescent (Fig 8). They are distributed throughout India, Sri Lanka and Burma (Matthew 1991).

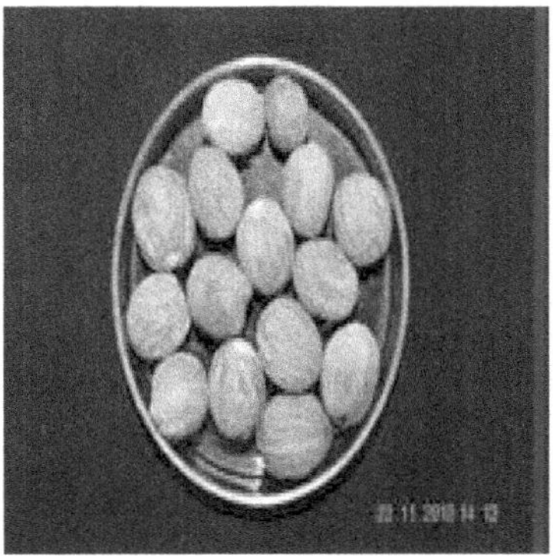

**Fig 8** The Dried Fruits Of *Terminalia bellirica* Used In KVC

In Siddha, the Fruit, leaf and seed are used in medicines. They cure Guinea worm disease, leucorrhoea, venereal diseases, hypertension, pox and dyspnoea (Yoganarasimhan, 2000).

(vii) *Phyllanthus emblica* L. *(Emblica officinalis* Gaertn,) (Euphorbiaceae)

*Phyllanthus emblica* plants are small deciduous trees with hairy reddish-brown branchlets. Their leaves are oblong, subsessile and distichous. The flowers are in axillary fascicles. The fruits are globose berries, 6-furrowed and greenish-yellow (Fig 9). They are distributed in the entire India, Indomalaysia, Sri Lanka and China (Matthew 1991).

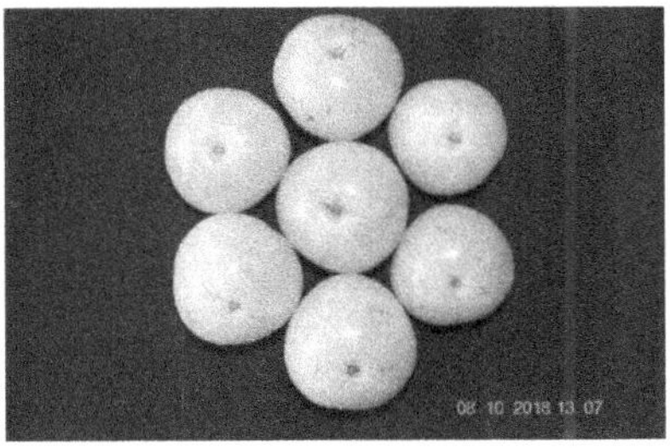

(a)

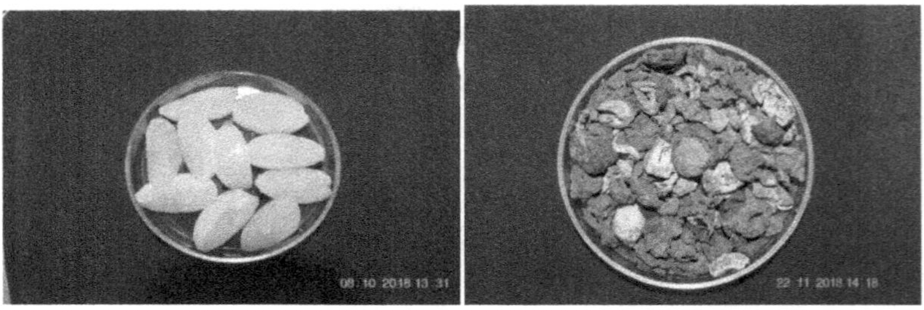

**(b)** **(c)**

**Fig 9** (a) The Fresh Fruits Of *Phyllanthus emblica,* (b) Sliced Fresh Fruits And (c) Shade Dried Fruits Used In KVC

The fruits are the useful parts. They are astringent, cooling, diuretic, laxative, and a rich source of vitamin C. In Siddha they are rejuvenators and are used in curing diseases of pittam, coryza, vomiting, constipation, fainting, polyuria, anaemia, ascites, piles, dropsy, hypertension, wasting diseases, asthma and tuberculosis (Yoganarasimhan, 2000).

(viii) *Salacia chinensis* L. (Celastraceae)

They are climbing shrubs or stragglers. Their leaves are elliptic-oblong, crenate and serrate. The flowers are greenish-yellow, 2 to 3 fascicled or on axillary tubercles. The fruits are globose berries, red when ripe. They are predominantly distributed in Dharmapuri, Salem, South Arcot, Thiruchchirappalli districts of Tamil Nadu, India and in Java, Sri Lanka and Philippines (Mathew, 1991).

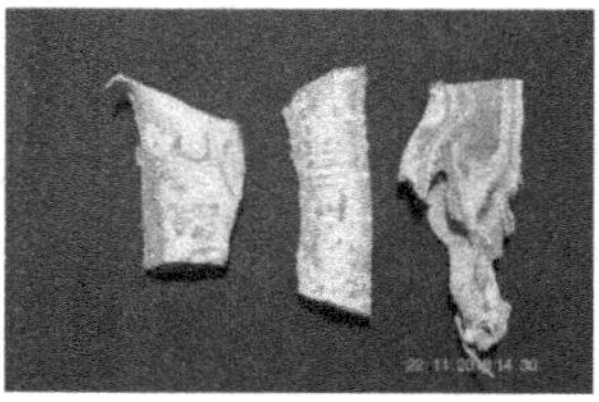

**Fig 10** The Dried Barks Of *Salacia chinensis* Used In KVC

The medicinally useful part of the plant is bark. The dried stem barks (Fig 10) are used in KVC. They are used in the drug preparation for diabetes and also used in abortifacient drugs. The bark decoction is given in amenorohoea, dysmenorrhoea, and venereal diseases. It is also used in alleviating kapha and pitha ( Yoganarasimhan, 2000).

### 4.2 Phytochemical and HPTLC Fingerprint Profile studies

#### 4.2a Phytochemical Analysis

The plant Kariveppilai Chooranan powder (25 g) was subjected to Soxhlet extraction process in a round bottom flask with ethanol (0.5 lts) for 12 h. The extract was concentrated under reduced pressure at 50-60°C till complete drying. The dried crude ethanolic extract of the plant (yield 3.79 g, 15.15 %) was stored in a closed vessel at 4°C.

**Detection for carbohydrates (Rosenthaler 1930)**

500 mg of extract was dissolved in 5 ml of distilled water and filtered. The filtrate was used to test the presence of carbohydrates.

**Molisch's test**:

Molish reagent: 10 gm of alpha napthol was dissolved in 100 ml of 95% methanol to prepare Molish reagent. To the extract, two drops of Molish reagent and few drops of concentrated $H_2SO_4$ was added. Formation of purple-violet ring indicates the presence of carbohydrates.

**Detection of Glycosides (Ronsenthaler, 1930; Sim, 1968)**

0.5 gm of the extract was hydrolyzed with 20 ml of HCl (0.1 N) and filtered. The filterate was used to test the presence of Glycosides.

**Keller-Killiani test:**

To the extract, a few drops of glacial acetic acid and one drop of 5% $FeCl_3$ and concentrated $H_2SO_4$ was added. Formation of reddish brown colour at the junction of two liquid layers and turned bluish green upper layer indicates the presence of glycosides.

**Detection of Saponins (Kokate, 2001)**

Foam test: 1 ml of extract was diluted to make up to 20 ml with distilled water and slowly shaked in a graduated cyclinder for 15 minutes. 1 one cm layer of foam indicates the presence of saponins.

**Detection of Alkaloids (Rosenthaler, 1930; Peach and Trancey, 1955)**

0.5 gm of the extract was dissolved in 10 ml of dilute HCl (0.1N) and filtered. The filterate was used to test the presence of alkaloids.

**Mayer's test**

Mayer's reagent is readily available from SD fine chemicals, Mumbai. Filtrate was treated with Meyer's reagent. Formation of yellow cream colored precipitate indicates the presence of alkaloids.

**Dragendrodroff's test**

Dragendroff's reagent is prepared by the following method:

i) Dissolve 8 gm of bismuth subnitrate in 20 ml of nitric acid.

ii) Dissolve 27.2 gm of Potassium iodide in 50 ml of distilled water, mix (a) and (b) and adjust the volume to 100 ml with distilled water. Filtrate was treated with

Dragendroff's reagent. Formation of red colored precipitate indicates the presenc of alkaloids.

**Detection of Flavonoids (Harbourne, 1973)**

**Alkaline reagent test**

To 100 mg of the extract, a few drops of NaOH solution was added in a test tube. Formation of intense yellow color that becomes colorless on addition of a few crops of of dilute HCl indicates the presence of flavonoids.

**Detection of Phenolics and Tannin (Ashtosh, 2004)**

100 mg of extract was boiled with 1 ml of distilled water and filtered. The filterate was used for the following tests,

**Ferric chloride test**

To a 2 ml of filtrate, 2 ml of 1% ferric chloride solution was added in a test tube. Formation of bluish black color indicates the presence of phenolic compounds.

**Test for Tannins:**

To the extract 0.5 ml NaOH was added. Formation of precipitate indicates the presence of tannins.

**Detection of Phytosterols and Triterpenoids (Peach and Tracy, 1955)**

0.5 gm of extract was treated with 10 ml chloroform and filtered. The filterate was used to test the presence of Phytosterols and Triterpenoids.

**Leibermann's test**

To a 2 ml of filtrate in hot alcohol, a few drops of acetic anhydride were added. Formation of brown precipitate indicates the presence of sterols.

**Leiberman-Bucharat test**

To the extract, a few drops of acetic acid and concentrated $H_2SO_4$ were added. Deep red ring at the junction of two layers indicates the presence of triterpenes.

**Salkowaski test**

To the extract solution, a few drops of conc. sulphuric acid was added and shaken and allowed to stand; lower layer turns red indicating the presence of sterols.

**Detection of fixed oils and fats (Rosenthaler, 1936)**

Oily spot test: One drop of extract was placed on filter paper and solvent was allowed to evaporate. An oily stain on filter paper indicates the presence of fixed oil and fat.

### 4.2b Determination of Moisture Content

About 5 g of each raw material were accurately weighed. The air dried material was taken in a previously dried and tared flat weighing bottle in IR moisture balance and the temperature was adjusted to 105°C and heating was done for 5 minutes. The procedure was repeated three times for different samples and the loss in weight was calculated with respect to the original weight. It gives the loss on drying (LOD).

The formula used for calculating LOD is = $(W1/W2) \times 100$

where, W1-weight of raw material after heating

W2- original weight of the raw material

### 4.2c Estimation of Extractive Values of Solvents

**Determination of chloroform soluble extractives**

5 g of air dried coarse powder of drugs was macerated with 100 ml of chloroform in a glass toppered conical flask with frequent shaking for 6 hours and then allowed to stand for 18 hours. Thereafter, it was filtered rapidly taking care against loss of solvent. About 25ml of the filtrate was evaporated in a tared flat-bottomed dish to dryness on water bath and then dried at 105$^0$C for 6 hours, cooled in a desiccator for 30 minutes and weighed immediately.

**Determination of water soluble extractives**

5 g of air dried coarse powder of drugs was macerated with 100 ml of water in a glass-stoppered conical flask with frequent shaking for 6 hours and then allowed to stand for 18 hours. Thereafter, it was filtered rapidly taking care against loss of solvent. About 25ml of the filtrate was evaporated in a tared flat-bottomed dish to dryness on water bath and then dried at $105^0$C for 6 hours, cooled in a desiccator for 30 minutes and weighed immediately.

**4.2d Determination of Ash Values**

Ash values (WHO, 1998) such as total ash, acid insoluble ash, and water soluble ash, acid soluble and sulfated ash were determined. The total ash determination method is designed to measure the total amount of material remaining after ignition. This includes both "physiological ash", which is derived from the plant tissue itself, and "non physiological ash", which is the residue of extraneous matter adhereing to the plant surface.

**Determination of Total ash**

About 3 g each of powdered parts were accurately weighed and taken separately in silica crucible, which was previously ignited and weighed. The powder was spread as a fine layer on the bottom of crucible. The powder was incinerated gradually by increasing temperature to make it dull red hot until free from carbon. The crucible was cooled and weighed. The procedure was repeated to get constant weight. The percentage of total ash was calculated with reference to the air dried powder.

**Acid insoluble ash**

The ash obtained as described above was boiled with 25 ml of 2N HCl for 5 minutes. The insoluble ash was collected on an ashless filter paper and washed with hot water. The insoluble ash was transferred into a crucible, ignited and weighed. The procedure was repeated to get a constant weight. The percentage of acid insoluble ash was calculated with reference to the air dried drug.

**Water soluble ash**

The ash obtained as described for the total ash was boiled for 5 minutes with 25 ml of water. The insoluble matter was collected on ashless filter paper and washed with hot water. The insoluble ash was transferred into silica crucible, ignited for 15 min. and weighed. The procedure was repeated to get a constant weight. The weight of insoluble matter was subtracted from the weight of total ash. The difference in weight was considered as water soluble ash. The percentage of water soluble ash was calculated with reference to air dried parts respectively.

**Acid soluble ash**

Total ash treated with dilute hydrochloric acid reacts with minerals to form soluble salts and the insoluble residue consists mainly of silica, as acid insoluble ash. To the crucible/silica dish containing the total ash obtained by the previous test, 25ml of HCl (N70g/l) was added, covered with a watch glass and boiled gently for 5 min on a hot plate or burner. Watch glass was rinsed with 5ml of hot water and washings were added to the crucible. Insoluble matter was collected on an ashless filter paper by filtration and rinsed repeatedly with hot water until the filtrate was found to be neutral/free from acid. Filter paper containing the insoluble matter was transferred to the original crucible, dried on a hot plate and ignited to a constant weight in the muffle furnace at 450°-500°C. Silica dish was allowed to cool in desiccator for 30 min and weighed without delay. Content of acid insoluble ash as % was calculated as given below:

Acid insoluble ash % = (B-C / A) × 100

Where, A = sample weight in g

B = wt. of dish + contents after drying (g)

C = wt. in g. of empty dish.

**Sulphated ash**

A silica crucible was heated to red for 10 min. and was allowed to cool in a desiccator and weighed. A one gram of substance was accurately weighed and transferred to the crucible. It was ignited gently at first, until the substance was thoroughly charred. Then the residue was cooled and moistened with 1 ml of concentrated sulphuric acid, heated gently until white fumes no longer evolved and ignited at 800°C ± 25°C until all black particles disappeared. The ignition was conducted in a place protected from air currents. The crucible was allowed to cool. A few drops of concentrated sulphuric acid was added and heated, ignited as before and was allowed to cool and weighed. The operation was repeated until two successive weighing do not differ by more than 0.5 mg.

**4.2e Biochemical Analysis**

**Preparation of the extract**

5gm of the drug was weighed accurately and placed in a 250ml clean beaker. 50ml of distilled water was added to this and dissolved well. Then it was boiled well for about 10 minutes, cooled and filtered in a 100ml volumetric flask and then it was made to 100ml with distilled water. This fluid was taken for analysis.

**4.2f HPTLC Fingerprint Profile Method**

**Sample preparation**

The test solution for the HPTLC (Yamunadevi, 2011) study was prepared by soaking 2.5gm of the drug (Karuvepillai Chooranam - Light Brown in color) in chloroform and kept overnight. The solution was boiled for 10 min and filtered. The filtrate was evaporated to dry ver a water bath. The dried solute was dissolved in chloroform and used as a test solution.

**HPTLC analysis**

Development of solvent system, sample application and documentation of the developed chromatograms was done as given below:

5μl and 10 μl of Chloroform extract of the test solution was spotted on the pre-coated silica gel 60 $F_{254}$ HPTLC plate (Merck) of uniform thickness 0.2mm using Linomat 5 sample applicator and developed in n-Hexane: Chloroform : Methanol (6.5:3.5:0.5). The loaded plate was visualized under UV light at 254nm and 366 nm using CAMAG REPROSTAR3 and chromatograms were photographed.

**Densitometry**

The plate was scanned at 254 nm using TLC Scanner and the finger print profiles were recorded.

## 4.3 Antioxidant Activity Studies

The test substance, KVC, was evaluated for *in vitro* antioxidant activity using ABTS with concentrations ranging from 100 μg ml to 6.25μg / ml, and DPPH and Nitric acid with concentration ranging from 1000μg/ml to 62.5μg/ml. The sample was evaluated for *in vitro* antioxidant activity against ABTS, DPPH and Nitric Oxide radicals (Sharma 2011).

### 4.3a ABTS Assay

**Preparation of test substance for ABTS assay**

Dissolve 21 mg of test substance in methanol separately to obtain solutions of 21 mg/ml concentration. Serially dilute this solution separately to obtain lower concentrations (6.25,12.5, 25, 50 and 100 μg/ml).

**Preparation of standard for ABTS assay**

Weigh 10 mg of Rutin and dissolve in 0.95 ml of methanol to get 10.5 mg/ml concentration. Serially dilute this solution with methanol to get lower concentrations (6.25, 12.5, 25, 50 and 100 μg/ml)

**ABTS inhibition Assay**

ABTS (5.48 mg) in 5 ml was dissolved in distilled water to get 2 mM concentration and potassium persulphate (17 mM, 0.03 ml) was added to the above. The reaction mixture was left to stand at room temperature overnight in dark before use and was prepared fresh for each trial. To 0.2 ml of various concentrations of the test substances or standards, 1.0 ml of PBS and 0.16 ml of ABTS solution were added to get a final volume of 1.36 ml in eppendorf tubes and cyclomixed. The same step was repeated for test blank and control blank, instead of ABTS reagent, 0.16 ml of distilled water was taken. After 20 minutes of incubation, 0.1 ml of reaction mixture was pipetted to microtiter plate in triplets for test, control and single for test blank and control blank. The absorbance in ELISA reader at 734 nm was measured and the values were recorded.

### 4.3b DPPH Assay

**Preparation of test substance for DPPH assay**

Dissolve 21 mg of test substance in DMSO separately to obtain solutions of 21 mg/ml concentration. Serially dilute these solutions separately to obtain lower concentrations (62.5,

125, 250, 500 and 1000 μg/ml) (Ali-Ismail, 2018, Saikrishna, 2013 and Miori Tanka *et al.* 2016).

**Preparation of standard for DPPH assay**

Weigh 10 mg of Quercetin or Ascorbic acid and dissolve in 0.95 ml of DMSO to get 10.5 mg/ml concentration. Serially dilute these solutions with DMSO to get lower concentrations (62.5, 125, 250, 500 and 1000 μg/ml).

**Antioxidant activity for DPPH radical**

The assay was carried out on a 96 well microtiter plate. 200μl of methanolic DPPH solution in triplets as test and control were taken and 200 μl of methanol for test blank and control blank in singlet were taken. 10 μl of each of the test substance or the standard from the lowest concentration was added and 10 μl DMSO serves as control and control blank. The plates were incubated at $370^0$C for 30 minutes and the absorbance of each solutions were measured at 490 nm, using ELISA reader.

**4.3c Nitric Oxide Radical Assay**

**Antioxidant activity for $NO_2$ radical**

Sodium nitroprusside (10 mM, 0.4 ml), phosphate buffer saline (PBS, pH 7.4, 0.1 ml) and 0.1ml of test substance or standard in DMSO of various concentrations were incubated at 25° C for 150 minutes. 0.1ml of DMSO was used for control and control blank. In place of sodium nitroprusside, distilled water was taken for test blank and control blank. Followed by incubation, 0.05 ml of the reaction mixture containing nitriteion was pipetted out from centrifuge tubes into microtiter plate in triplets for test and control. Control blank and test blank were taken in singlet. 0.1 ml of sulphanilic acid reagent was added to all the wells, mixed and allowed to stand for 5 min for completion of diazotization. Then, 0.1 ml of NEDD was added and allowed to stand for 30 minutes in diffused light. The absorbance of these solutions was measured at 540 nm using ELISA reader.

## 4.4 Antimicrobial and Antiadipogenesis Studies

### 4.4a *In vitro* antibacterial activity

**Preparation of Sample for Experimental Work**

10 gm of the homogenized drug sample was taken aseptically and dissolved in 10 ml of sterile water and made up to 100 ml with the sterile water. The insoluble drug product was suspended in 100 ml of buffered sodium chloride-peptone solution (pH 7.0).

**Serial dilution of the sample**

Serial dilution is the dilution of a sample, in 10-fold dilutions. From the sample, 1 ml was added to 9 ml of sterile distilled water and mixed well. This dilution was denoted as $10^{-1}$ dilution. From this dilution, 1 ml was taken from that mixture and is added to 9 ml, and designated as $10^{-2}$ dilution. The same procedure was repeated up to $10^{-4}$.

**Isolation of Bacteria by Plate Count Method**

In this test, the bacterial sample was made to grow as colonies, by inoculating a known volume of sample into a solidifiable nutrient medium (Nutrient agar medium) in petridish. The agar plate was prepared by mixing growth medium with agar and then sterilized by autoclaving. Once the agar was cooled to 45°C, approximately 15 to 20 ml of medium was poured into a sterile petri dish under aseptic condition in a laminar air flow chamber and left to solidify for 15 minutes. After solidification, each plate was smeared with 0.1 ml of sample from the dilution of $10^{-1}$ and $10^{-2}$. After inoculation, all the plates were incubated at 37°C for 24 hours. After incubation, the bacterial colonies developed were visible to the naked eye and the number of colonies on a plate was counted using Quebec Colony Counter. Plates with an average of 30 to 300 colonies of the target bacterium were selected for colony count. Plates with lower than 30 colonies and greater than 300 colonies were rejected.

**Composition of Nutrient Agar Media**

| | |
|---|---|
| Peptone | : 5.0 gm |
| Sodium chloride | : 5.0 gm |
| Beef extract | : 1.5 gm |
| Yeast extract | : 1.5 gm |
| Agar | : 15.0 gm |
| Distilled water | : 1000 ml |
| pH ( at 25°C) | : 7.4±0.2 |

**Evaluation of Antimicrobial Activity of Drug**

Antimicrobial activity was performed by agar well diffusion method on agar.

**Preparation of drug extracts solution for the experiment**

The KVC powder was weighed and dissolved in sterile distilled water to prepare appropriate dilution to get required concentrations of about 10, 20 and 30µg/ml. They were kept under refrigerated condition until they were used for the experiment.

**Procedure for the Agar Well Diffusion Test**

The antibacterial screening of the drugs was carried out by determining the zone of inhibition using agar well diffusion method. All the drug extracts were tested against four pathogenic bacterial strains of gram positive and gram negative organism by agar well diffusion method.

**Bacterial Inoculum Preparation**

Inoculum of *Staphylococcus aureus*, *Escherichia coli*, *Klebsiella pneumoniae*, *Proteus vulgaris*, and *Bacillus substilis* were prepared in nutrient broth medium and kept for incubation at 37°C for 8 hrs.

**Agar well-diffusion method**

This method was followed to determine the antimicrobial activity. Muller-Hinton Agar media plates were swabbed (sterile cotton swabs) with 8 hour old broth culture of respective bacteria. After inoculation, wells with the size of 10 mm diameter and about 2 cm apart were made in each of these plates using sterile cork borer. Stock solution of each drug extract was prepared at a concentration of 1 mg/ml in water. About 100 μl of different concentrations of drug solvent extracts were added into the wells and allowed to diffuse at room temperature for 2 hrs. The plates were incubated at 37°C for 24 hrs. After incubation, the diameter of the inhibition zone (mm) was measured and the activity index was also calculated.

**Composition of Muller Hinton Agar Media**

| | |
|---|---|
| Beef Extract | : 02.00 gm |
| Acid Hydrolysate of Casein | : 17.50 gm |
| Starch | : 01.50 gm |
| Agar | : 17.00 gm |

**Components of Eosin Methylene Blue Agar Media**

| | |
|---|---|
| Pancreatic digest of gelatin | : 10.0 g |
| Dibasic potassium phosphate | : 2.0 g |
| Lactose | : 10.0 g |

| | |
|---|---|
| Eosin Y | : 400 mg |
| Methylene blue | : 65 mg |
| Agar | : 15.0 g |
| Distilled water | : 1000 ml |

**Evaluation of Specified Microorganisms**

**Isolation and Identification of *Escherichia coli***

One ml of the prepared sample was added in a sterile screw-capped container containing 50 ml of nutrient broth and mixed well. Then, it was allowed to stand for 1 hour and mixed well again. After one hour, the screw caps of the bottle was loosened and incubated at 37° for 18 to 24 hours.

**Primary Test**

From the above prepared enrichment culture, 1.0 ml was taken and transferred aseptically into a tube containing 5 ml of Mac Conkey broth. Inoculated tubes were incubated in a water-bath at 36° to 38° for 48 hours.

**Secondary Test**

From the primary test, 1.0 ml of the enrichment culture was taken and transferred aseptically in to 5 ml of peptone water. It was then incubated in a water-bath at 43.5° C to 44.5° C for 24 hours and observed the tubes for acid and gas. Then, the culture was subjected to biochemical tests and results were observed and correlated.

**Alternative test**

It was done by a loop-full of enriched culture in the primary test streaked on a sterile Mac Conkey agar medium. Then, the plates were inverted and incubated at 37 ° C for 24 hours. After incubation, the pink or brick red color colonies were examined and transferred individually into the surface of Eosin Methylene Blue agar medium (EMB), on Petri dishes. Inoculated plates were inverted and incubated at 37 ° C for 24 hours. After incubation, the colonies on medium were checked for their color appearance like green metallic sheen under reflected light. The colonies were subjected to confirmation by further suitable cultural and biochemical tests.

**Isolation and Identification of *Salmonella* sp.**

1 ml of the prepared sample was added in a sterile screw-capped container containing 100 ml of nutrient broth and mixed well. Then, it was allowed to stand for 1 hour and mixed well again. After one hour, the screw caps of the bottle was loosened and incubated at 37°C for 18 to 24 hours.

**Primary Test**

From the above prepared enrichment culture, 1.0 ml was taken and transferred aseptically into a tube containing 10 ml of Selenite F broth. Inoculated tubes were incubated in a water-bath at 36°C to 38°C for 48 hours. After incubation, the culture was subcultured on two of the agar media, namely, bismuth sulphate agar and deoxycholate citrate agar and incubated the plates at 36°C to 38°C for 18 to 24 hours. After incubation, colonies were observed on the medium and confirmed the genus *Salmonella* based on guidelines.

**Secondary test**

The suspected colonies of the primary test were subcultured on the slant of triple sugar-iron agar in test tube and in urea broth. Both media were incubated at 37°C for 24 hours. After incubation, the results were observed according to the development of color change and acid / gas in media. The presence of *Salmonella* was confirmed by agglutination tests.

**Composition of *Salmonella Shigella* Agar Media**

| | |
|---|---|
| Beef Extract | : 5.0 gm |
| Enzymatic Digest of Casein | : 2.5 g |
| Enzymatic Digest of Animal Tissue | : 2.5 gm |
| Lactose | : 10 gm |
| Bile salts | : 8.5 gm |
| Sodium Citrate | : 8.5 gm |
| Ferric Citrate | : 1.0 gm |
| Brilliant Green | : 0.00033 gm |
| Neutral Red | : 0.025 |
| Agar | : 13.5 gm |
| Distilled water | : 1000 ml |

**Isolation and Identification of *Pseudomonas aeruginosa***

From the above prepared enrichment culture, 1.0 ml was taken and transferred aseptically into 100 ml of fluid soyabean-casein digest medium and mixed well. The inoculated tubes were incubated at 37° C for 24 hours. After incubation, the growth of bacteria was checked. From this, a loop-full of culture was streaked on the surface of Cetrimide agar medium and *Pseudomonas* Isolation Agar medium and incubated at incubated at 37° C for 24 hours. After incubation, the colonies from the agar surface of these two media were checked for detection of fluorescein and pyocyanin.

**Composition of Cetrimide Agar Media**

| | |
|---|---|
| Pancreatic digest of gelatin | : 20.0 g |
| Magnesium chloride | : 1.4 g |
| Potassium sulphate | : 10.0 g |
| Cetrimide | : 0.3 g |
| Agar | : 13.6 g |
| Glycerin | : 10.0 g |
| Distilled Water | : 1000 ml |

**Isolation and Identification of *Staphylococcus aureus***

From the above prepared enrichment culture, a loop full of culture was taken and transferred aseptically on Mannitol salt agar and incubated at 37° C for 24 hours.. After incubation, the colonies were subjected to confirmation by hem agglutination test.

**Composition of Mannitol Salt Agar Media**

| | |
|---|---|
| Pancreatic digest of gelatin | : 5.0 g |
| Peptic digest of animal tissue | : 5.0 g |
| Beef extract | : 1.0 g |
| D-Mannitol | : 10.0 g |
| Sodium chloride | : 75.0 g |
| Agar | : 15.0 g |
| Phenol red | : 25 mg |
| Distilled Water | : 1000 ml |

### 4.4b *In vitro* Antifungal Activity

In order to access the biological significance and ability of the sample, the antifungal activity was determined by Agar well diffusion method. The antifungals present in the samples are allowed to diffuse out into the medium and interact in a plate freshly seeded with the test organisms. The resulting zones of inhibition will be uniformly circular as there will be a confluent lawn of growth. The diameter of zone of inhibition can be measured in millimeters.

**Materials required**

1) Potato Dextrose Agar Medium (1 L)

The medium was prepared by dissolving 39 g of the commercially available Potato Dextrose Agar Medium (HiMedia) in 1000ml of distilled water. The dissolved medium was autoclaved at 15 lbs pressure at 121°C for 15 minutes. The autoclaved medium was mixed well and poured onto 100mm petriplates (25-30ml/plate) while still molten.

3. Clotrimazole (standard antifungal agent, concentration: 10mg / ml)

4. Culture of test organisms; growth of culture adjusted according to McFarland Standard, 0.5%

- *Aspergillus niger* (ATCC 16404)
- *Candida albicans*(ATCC 10231)

**PROCEDURE**

**Isolation of Fungi**

From each of the above prepared samples, 0.1 ml of sample was transferred to Sabouraud Dextrose agar (SDA) prepared with Chloramphenicol. The plates were then incubated for 5 days at room temperature (20 to 25°C). After incubation, the fungal colonies were observed and calculated.

Composition of SDA

| | |
|---|---|
| Dextrose | ; 40 gm |
| Peptone | : 10 gm |
| Agar | : 15 gm |
| Distilled water | : 1000 ml |

Potato Dextrose Agar plates were prepared and overnight grown species of fungus, *Aspergillus niger and Candida albicans* were swabbed. Wells of approximately 10mm was bored using a well cutter and samples of different concentrations such as 250µg/mL, 500µg/mL and 1000µg/mL were added. The zone of inhibition was measured after overnight incubation at room temperature and compared with that of standard antimycotic (Clotrimazole) **(NCCLS, 1993).**

### 4.4c *In vivo* Hypolipidemic Activity

**Materials and Methods**

Wister albino rats were obtained from central animal house, K.M.College of Pharmacy, Madurai, Tamil Nadu. The animals were given standard rodent diet and water ad libitum throughout the study. The rats used in the present study were maintained in accordance with the guidelines of the National Institute of Nutrition, Indian Council for Medical Research, Hyderabad, India and the study was approved by Institutional Animal Ethical Committee, Government Siddha Medical College, Palayamkottai (Given in Annexure).

**Materials:**

- Herbal Siddha formulation of Karivepillai Chooranam (KVC)
- Cholesterol extra pure for feeding purpose was obtained from S D fine-chem. Limited, Mumbai, India. Coconut oil was used as a vehicle for cholesterol feeding.
- Atorvastatin was obtained from Micro labs, Bangalore, India.

**Experimental procedure:**

All the animals were weighed and divided into five groups each of six animals.

Group I : Normal control.

Group II : Cholesterol control. Fed cholesterol at a dose of 400mg/kg body weight for 30 days.

Group III: Feed cholesterol as in group II and Atorvastatin 1mg/kg body weight from day 15 to day 30 **(Vijaya, 2009)**

Group IV : Feed cholesterol as in group II and herbal Siddha formulation of Karuveppilaichooranam at a dose of 100mg/kg body weight from day 15 to day 30.

Group V : Feed cholesterol as in group II and herbal siddha formulation of KVC at a dose of 200mg/kg body weight from day 15 to day 30.

At the end of 30 days, all the rats were sacrificed, blood was collected, allowed to clot and serum was obtained by centrifugation. The serum samples were used for various biochemical procedures.

**Biochemical analysis**

The serum was analyzed for total cholesterol, triglycerides, high density lipoprotein (HDL), low density lipoprotein (LDL), very low density lipoprotein (VLDL), by using standard protocol methods (Auto Analyzer).

environmental condition of temperature ($22^0C \pm 5^0C$) and humidity (55 ±5%) and 12 hr light dark cycles throughout the experimental period.

**Induction of diabetes mellitus**

Diabetes mellitus was induced in wistar rats by single intraperitoneal injection of freshly prepared solution of Streptozotocin (25mg/kg BW) in physiological saline after overnight fasting for 12hrs (Al-Shamaony 1994).

Streptozotocin is commonly used to produce diabetes mellitus in experimental animals due to its ability to destroy the β-cells of pancreas possibly by generating the excess reactive oxygen species such as $H_20_2$, $0_2$ and $H0^-$. The development of hyperglycemias in rats is confirmed by plasma glucose estimation 72 hrs post Streptozotocin injections. The rats with fasting plasma glucose level of >180-220mg/dl were used for this experiment.

**Experimental procedure:**

In the experiment, a total of 30 rats (24 diabetic surviving rats & 6 normal rats) were used. Diabetes was induced in rats 3 days before starting the experiment. The rats were divided into 5 groups after the induction of Streptozotocin diabetes. In the experiment 6, rats were used in each group.

**Study design**

Group I: Normal (control) consists of normal rats which were given with 10ml/Kg of normal saline orally.

Group II: Toxic (control) Diabetic rats which received 25mg/Kg of Streptozotocin through I.P.

GroupIII: Diabetic rats which received glipizide at a dose of (10mg/Kg orally) for 28 days.

Group IV: Diabetic rats whcih received KARUVEPPILAI CHOORANAM at a dose of (100mg/Kg orally) for 28 days.

Group V : Diabetic rats which received KVC at a dose of (200mg/Kg orally) for 28 days.

**Methodology**

**Sample collection:**

After 28 days of treatment, body weight, blood glucose, haemoglobin, glycosylated haemoglobin, plasma insulin, total cholesterol, triglycerides, HDL-cholesterol and phospholipids and glycogen content and antioxidant enzymes level were determined. Blood was collected from the eyes (venous pool) by sino-ocular puncture **(Wayen 1980)** in EDTA coating plasma tubes for the estimation of blood parameters.

**Biochemical Analysis**

**Estimation of blood glucose:**

Blood glucose was estimated by commercially available glucose kit (One Touch Ultra) Johnson based on glucose oxidase method (Trinder 1969)

**Plasma insulin:**

Plasma insulin was determined by ELISA method using a Boehringer–Mannheim kit (Anderson 1993) with an ES300 Boehringer analyzer (Mannheim, Germany).

**Estimation of total haemoglobin and glycosylated haemoglobin:**

Total haemoglobin was determined by the method of Drabkin and Austin, (1932) and glycosylated haemoglobin was determined by the method of Sudhakar Nayak and Pattabiraman (1981).

**Estimation of lipid & lipoprotein:**

Plasma lipids were determined by auto analyzer according to the method of Total Choloterol (Parkeh and Jung, 1970) HDL-cholesterol (Gidez and Webb, 1950) phospholipids (Zilver, 1950) triglycerides (Rice, 1970).

**Hepatic glucokinase and hexokinase activity**

The part of liver for each test was perfused with ice cold 0.15M KCl and 1mm EDTA solution and homogenized twice its weight of ice cold buffer (0.01 cysteine and 1mm EDTA in 0.1 ml Tris-HCl, pH 7.4), and centrifuged for 20 min at $4^0$C. Glucose phosphorylation was assayed by means of glucose 6 phosphate dependent spectrophotometric method (Crane *et al.,* 1955).

**Glucose-6-phosphatase activity**

The part of the liver for each test was homogenized with 40 times its weight of ice cold buffer (0.1 citrate-KOH, pH 6.5) and filtered through cheese cloth. Glucose-6-phosphatase activity was measured by phosphate release by the method Marjorie. The determination of phosphoric acid concentration in assay mixture was done colorimetrically (Fiske *et al.* 1925).

**Glycogen Content**

The tissue sample was digested by hot concentrated 30% KOH and treated with anthrone reagent. Glycogen content was determined colorimetrically (Morales *et al.*, 1973).

**Statistical analysis**

The data for various biochemical parameters were analyzed using analysis of variance (ANOVA), and the group means were compared by Newman-Keul's multiple range test (NMKT). The values were considered statistically significant at $p<0.01$.

### 4.5c Antidiabetic Activity using $L_6$ Cell Line study

**Preparation of test solution**

The test drugs KVC was separately dissolved in DMSO and volume was made up with DMEM-HG supplemented with 2% inactivated FBS to obtain a stock solution of 10 mg/ml concentration and sterilized by filtration. Serial two fold dilutions were prepared from this for carrying out cytotoxic studies.

**Cell line and Culture medium**

Cell lines L-6 (Rat skeletal muscle) was cultured in DMEM-HG media supplemented with 10% inactivated Fetal Bovine Serum (FBS), penicillin (100 IU/ml), streptomycin (100μg/ml) and amphotericin B (5μg/ml) in a humidified atmosphere of 5% $CO_2$ at 37°C until confluent. The cells were dissociated with TPVG solution (0.2% trypsin, 0.02% EDTA, 0.05% glucose in PBS). The stock cultures were grown in 25 $cm^2$ culture flasks and all the experiments were carried out in 96 well microtitre plates.

## 4.6 Cytotoxicity and Heavy Metal Analysis

### 4.6a Acute Toxicity Study

**Outline of the method**

The in-vitro cytotoxicity was performed for test extract on Mouse Embryo Fibroblast cells to find out the toxic concentration of KVC. Based on this concentration, the adipogenesis activity of KVC by Oil Red O staining and free triglyceride level was measured.

**Preparation of test Solution**

For cytotoxicity studies, 10mg test drug was separately dissolved in DMSO and volume was made up with DMEM - high glucose supplemented with 2% inactivated FBS to obtain a stock solution of 1 mg/ml concentration and sterilized by 0.22μ syringe filtration. Serial two fold dilutions were prepared from this for carrying out cytotoxicity studies.

## SEM ANALYSIS

A scanning electron microscope (SEM) scans focused electron beam over a surface to create an immage. The electrons in the beam interact with the sampleprocucing various signals that can be used to ontain information about the surface topographyand composition,it is used for micro analysis of inorganic substances.KVCwas undergone this study and found material shape and size

## 4.7 Clinical Trial Study

**The open labeled single blind non randomized control study**

The clinical study was conducted at Government Siddha Medical College, Palayankottai, Tirunelveli, Tamil Nadu. The patients were selected after careful selection by include and excluded criteria. The clinical study was approved by IEC committee, A total of forty patients, twenty out patients and twenty in patients were treated for a total a period 3 months. The history of patients was noted before and after treatment.

# RESULTS AND DISCUSSION

# 5. RESULTS AND DISCUSSION

## 5.1 Phytochemical and HPTLC Fingerprint Profile Studies

### 5.1a Results of Phytochemical analysis

The medicinal value of these plants lie in some chemical bioactive substances that produce a definite physiological action on the human body. The most important of these bioactive constituents of plants are alkaloids, tannins, flavonoids and phenolic compounds (Edeogal, et.al 2005, Irshad 2002). The Phytochemical screening of the alcohol and aqueous extracts of plant samples revealed the presence of glycosides, alkaloids, flavonoids and tannins in all the plant extracts (Table 2). The following results were found in aqueous extract of Kariveppillai choornam.

Aqueous extract of Karivepillaichooranam contained carbohydrates, Glycosides, Alkaloids, phenolic, Terpenoids, Saponins, Flavonoids and Tannin compounds. The above phytochemical components are very important to reduce free radicals (Chitra, 2002) and the importance of individual phytochemical is described in below,

### Activity Of Phenolic Acids

The biological activities of phenolic acids are related increase bile secretion. reduce time of blood cholesterol and lipid levels (Arora ,2000) and anti microbial activity against bacteria, especialy *Straphylococcus aureus*. Phenolic acids are biologicaly acting as antiulcer, anti-inflammatory, antioxidant (Ghasemi 2009), cytotoxic and antitumor activities (MamtaSaxena,2013). Phenolic acids are reduced or act against oxidative damage leading to various degenerative diseases and have higher leves of reactive oxygen species (ROS) than normal cells.

**Table 2.** The Results Of Various Tests Of Phytochemical Analysis Of KVC

| Test | Observation | Inference |
|---|---|---|
| **Sample Code : Aqueous Extract** | | |
| **1.** Alkaloids | An orange red precipitate produced | Presence of Alkaloids |
| **2.** Flavanoids | A reddish pink or dirty brown colour was produced | Presence of Flavanoids |
| **3.** Saponins | A honey comb like froth was formed | Presence of Saponins |
| **4.** Phenols | A blue or green colour was formed. | Presence of Phenols |
| **5.** Steroids | A red color was produced in the chloroform layer. | Presence of Steroids |
| **6.** Glycosides | A yellow colour was formed. | Presence of Glycosides |
| **7.** Terpenoids | A red colour was formed on the chloroform layer. | Presence of Terpenoids |
| **8.** Tannins | Bluish- black colour disappeared on the addition of Sulphuric acid. | Presence of Tannins |

Therapeutics effect of polyphenol is good antioxidant, The metabolism regulator and antiangiogenic effects of KVCwere found increase in phase II detoxifying and antioxidant enzymes like HO-GST by modulation transcription factor Nrf 2, the curcumin protects against neuronal degeneration by reducing ROS neutralizing NO induced free radicals. Secondry metabolities of polyphenols like Procyanidins, Reveratrol and anthocyanin have Anti inflammatory effect via decreased expiration of iNOS and COX-2 inhibit inflammatory phenomenon. Phenolic compounds, namely, chlorogenic acid (CGA) and ferulic acid are considered as potent anti diabetic agent, pharmacologicaly phenolic compounds were known to enhance the uptake of 2DG in time and it was significantly upregulate the expression of GULT4 and PPAR-y and PK13K expression (Swapna Upadhyay and Madhulika Dixit 2015).

**Activity Of Tannin**

Activity of tannin is commonly used as astrigents with antiseptic, antioxidant and haemostatic action. The biological action of tannin is a potential metal ion chelators, protein precipitating agents, biological antioxidant and prevention of cellular oxidative damage including lipid peroxidation (Anila and Vijayalakshmi,2002).

**Activity Of Terpenoids**

Functional derivatives of terpenoids (Lycopene, Lutein, Abscorbic acid) are anti-inflammatory with good antioxidative activity (Okwu,2005) via significantly increased antioxidant enzymes SOD, GSH-PX, GR and GSH levels and lycopene reduce MDA levels (Conti, 1991) increase GSH levels in post menopausal woman and protects cardio vascular diseases. Lycopene reduces proinflammatory cytokine TNF-X by decreased NF-KB activation. So, these is significant inhibition of lipid peroxidation.

**Activity Of Saponins**

Saponins are known for their most beneficial effects on blood cholesterol levels, cancer, bone strenth and stimulate the immune system. Saponins bind with bile salt and cholesterol in the intestinal tract. Bile salts from small micelles with cholesterol facilitate its absorption. Saponins cause a reduction of blood cholesterol by preventing its re-absorption. The non sugar part of saponins have also a direct antioxidant activity, which may results in other benefits such as reduced risk of cancer and heart diseases (Mamta Saxena *et al.*, 2016).

**Activity Of Flavonoids**

The biological activity of flavonoids is antimicrobial, anti-inflammatory, oesterogenic, vascular and antitumor activities (Block *et al.*,1992 and Willet, 2002). The capacity of flavonoids to act as antioxidants depends upon their molecular structure. The position of hydroxyl groups and other feature in the chemical structure of flavonoids are an important role as an antioxidant with free radical scavenging activities (Vaya *et al.*, 2003, Way and Lee 2004). Flavonoids play a major role in protecting biological systems against the harmful effects of oxidative processes on macromolecules, such as carbohydrates, proteins, lipids and DNA.

*In vitro* flavonoids study proved them to be enzyme inhibitors (Histidine decarboxylase and Hyaluronidase), Hyaluronidase is a strengthen the inter cellular ground substances in the perivascular sheath. Flavonoids are non specific inhibitior of catechol-methyl transferase with its increased availability leading to a decrease in vascular fragility and anti-platelet aggregation activity.

Several flavonoids cirsiliol and hypolaetin are potent inhibitiors of the Lipogenase, inhibiting cyclooxygenase and platelet aggregation. The derived flavonols (quercetin, kaemferol and Myricetin) have been reported to exhibit various biological functions and medicinal properties such as antioxidant antithrombotic, anti-inflammatory, antiatherogenic and antiatherosclrotic with cardio protective effects (Taskinen and Belz.,1986; Taskinen., 2002).

So, the Kariveppillai choornam contain flavonoids, which have been proven to significantly lower the risk of hyperlipidemia and coronary vascular disease.

The following tests are used for the analysis of phytochemicals as described by (Harborne., 1973) they were carried out on alcoholic extract of KVC.

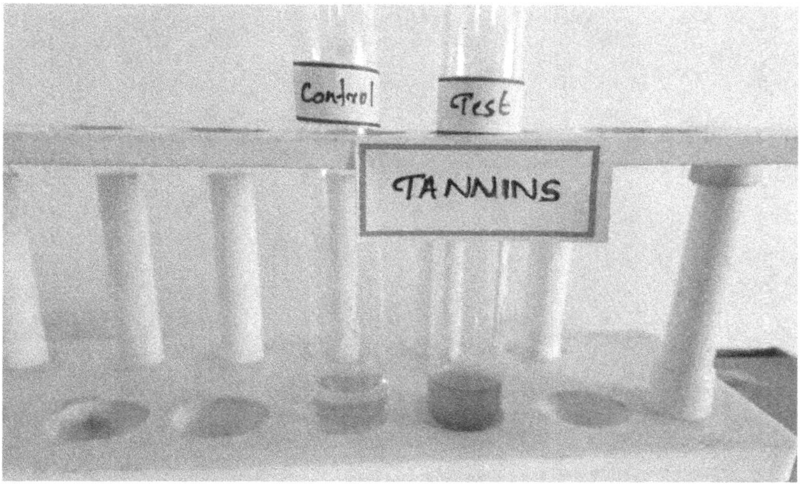


**Fig 11** Test of Tannin

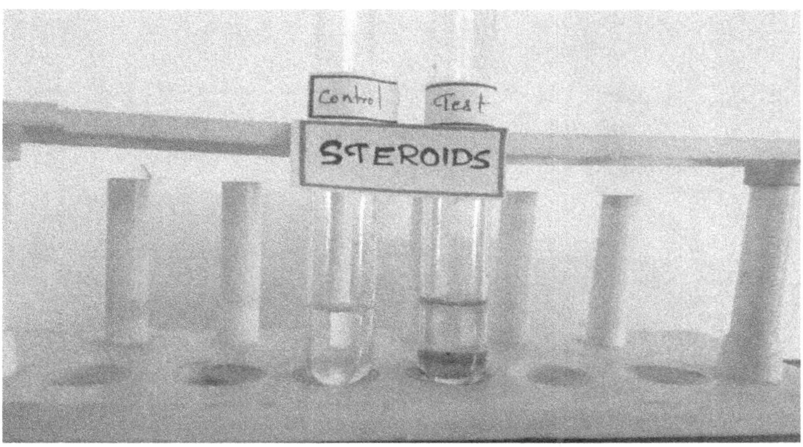


**Fig 12** Test of Strereoids

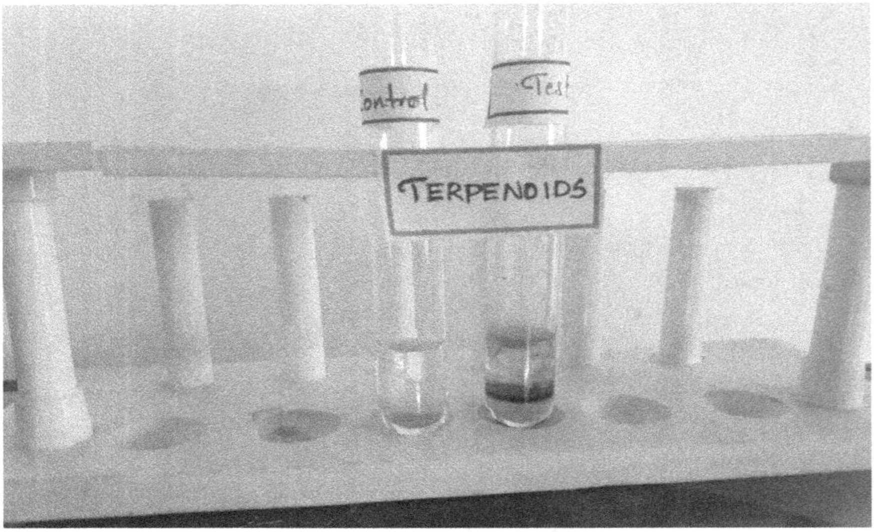


**Fig 13** Test of Terpenoids

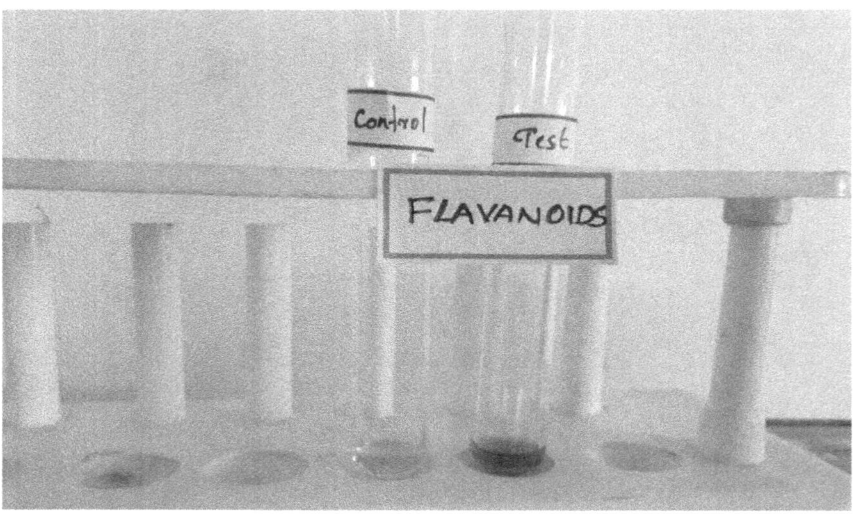


**Fig 14** Test of Flavanoids

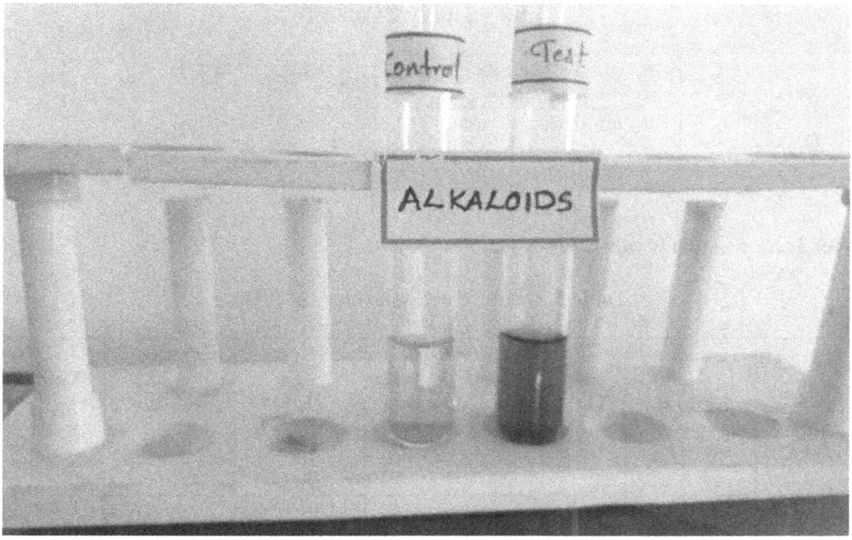


**Fig 15** Test of Alkaloids

**Extraction and Pharmacognosy analysis:**

As per the Table 3 Ethanolic extract of Karivepillaichooranam was 15.15%. In the case of chloroform, the extract value was 22.4% and for aqueous it was 21.64% .

**Table 3** Extractive Values Of KVC In Different Solvents

| S.No | Solvents | Percentage of Extract (w/w) |
|---|---|---|
| 1 | Ethanol | 15.15% |
| 2 | Chloroform Extract | 22.40% |
| 3 | Aqueous Extract | 21.64% |

As per the Table 4 Moister content of KVC was found to be 8.2%.

**Table 4** Moisture Content

| Test sample | Moisture content |
|---|---|
| Karivepillai choornam | 8.2 % |

As per Table 5 explains valuse for KVC.

**Table 5** The different Ash values of KVC

| **S.No** | **Sample** | **Total Ash** | **Acid Insoluble Ash (%)** | **Acid Soluble Ash (%)** | **Water Soluble Ash (%)** | **Sulfated Ash (%)** |
|---|---|---|---|---|---|---|
| 1 | Powdered plant-Drug | 5.36 | 1.20 | 14.93 | 16.70 | 1.95 |

foreign mater was Nil and loss on drying at 110°c yeilded a total ash value of 5.36% with acid in soluble ash 1.20%, acid soluble ash 14.93%, water soluble ash 16.70% and Sulfated ash 1.95%.

The Phytochemical compounds which occur naturally in plants are responsible for color and biological properties. The plant chemicals and antioxidant components are (Endogenous (or) Exogenous) interact and synergistically to neutralize the free radicals (Mark, 1998). The term is generally used to refer to those chemicals that may have biological significance but are not established as essential nutrients.

## 5.1b Results of HPTLC, Fingerprint Profile studies

HPTLC fingerprint profile were recorded for the KVC. The HPTLC image of KVC extract under UV 254 nm and under UV 366 nm is shown in Fig 16.

The KVC shows three major spots under UV at 254 nm (Fig 16) and under UV at 366 nm . eight major spots are formed (Fig 16) . The 3D densitometry chromatogram developed using 5 μl and 10 μl of test solution shows similar peaks (Fig 17).

HPTLC fingerprint profile of 5 μl test solution show eight major peak at Rf values 0.4, 0.09, 0.13, 0.19, 0.38, 0.43, 0.60 and 0.89. The heigst peak area was found at the Rf value of 0.89 with maximum peak area of 55000.9 (74.42) (Fig 18 and Table 7).

The major peaks are at Rf value 0.04, 0.09, 0.13, 0.60, and 0.89 indicating the presents of the phyto chemicals. The 10 μl test solution show at seven major peaks at Rf values of 0.03, 0.08, 0.11, 0.16, 0.41, o.52 and 0.85 with highest peak area at Rf value of 0.85 with 84211.4 (75.60%) (Fig 19 and Table 8).

**HPTLC Fingerprinting Profile Of KVC Of Based On Terpenoids Under UV**

PHOTO DOCUMENTATION UNDER UV

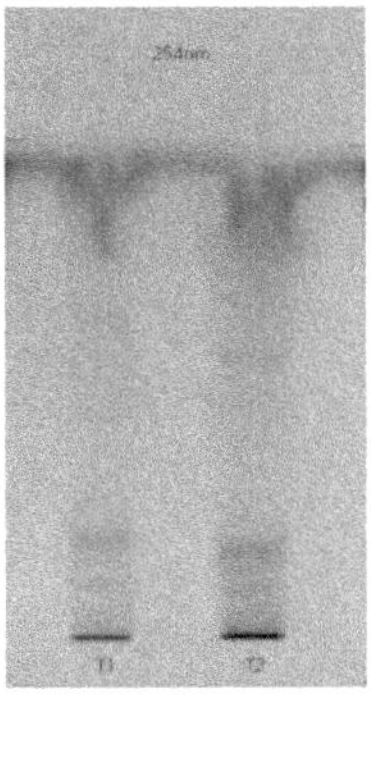

**T1- 5μl T2 -10μl**

**Fig 16a**

**AT 254nm**

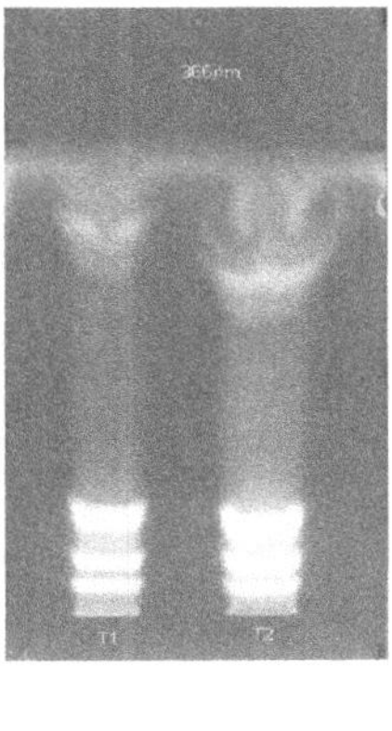

**T1-5μ l T2-10μl**

**Fig 16b**

**AT 366nm**

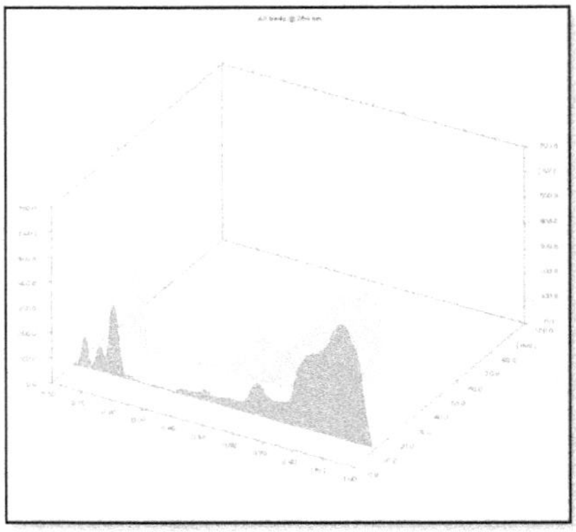

**Fig 17** 3D densimetry chromatogram of KVC at 254nm

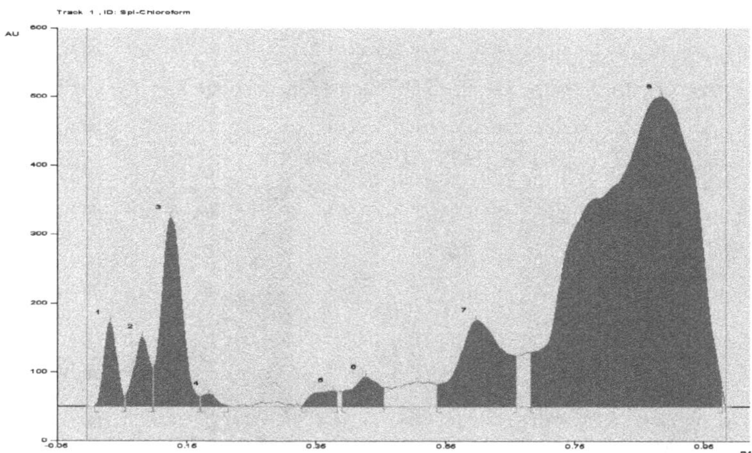


**Fig 18** HPTLC Fingerprint profile with peak display for 5μl test solution of KVC at 254nm

**Table 7** The Rf value for 5µl of alcohol extract of KVC at 254nm

| Peak | Start Rf | Start Height | Max Rf | Max Height | Height % | End Rf | End Height | Area | Area % |
|---|---|---|---|---|---|---|---|---|---|
| 1 | 0.01 | 0.4 | 0.04 | 120.9 | 10.49 | 0.06 | 14.2 | 1802.8 | 2.44 |
| 2 | 0.06 | 14.9 | 0.09 | 100.4 | 8.71 | 0.10 | 55.5 | 1811.7 | 2.45 |
| 3 | 0.10 | 56.9 | 0.13 | 273.5 | 23.72 | 0.17 | 14.0 | 6353.6 | 8.60 |
| 4 | 0.18 | 14.4 | 0.19 | 17.9 | 1.55 | 0.22 | 1.3 | 310.3 | 0.42 |
| 5 | 0.33 | 0.2 | 0.38 | 22.8 | 1.98 | 0.39 | 21.1 | 635.7 | 0.86 |
| 6 | 0.40 | 22.0 | 0.43 | 42.3 | 3.67 | 0.46 | 27.6 | 1374.0 | 1.86 |
| 7 | 0.54 | 31.6 | 0.60 | 125.2 | 10.86 | 0.67 | 73.4 | 6613.9 | 8.95 |
| 8 | 0.69 | 78.2 | 0.89 | 450.0 | 39.02 | 0.98 | 26.2 | 55003.9 | 74.42 |

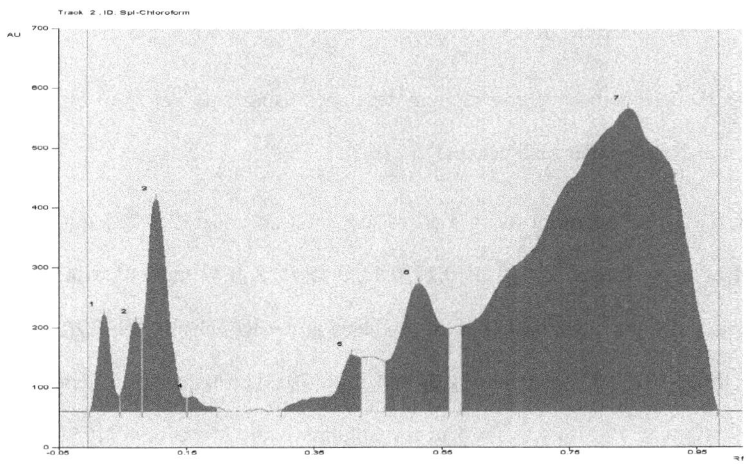


**Fig 19** HPTLC Fingerprint profile with peak display for 10µl test solution of KVC at 254nm

**Table 8** The Rf value for 10μl of alcohol extract of KVC at 254nm

| eak | Start Rf | Start Height | Max Rf | Max Height | Height % | End Rf | End Height | Area | Area % |
|---|---|---|---|---|---|---|---|---|---|
| 1 | 0.00 | 0.2 | 0.03 | 162.3 | 10.78 | 0.05 | 25.3 | 2491.7 | 2.24 |
| 2 | 0.05 | 26.9 | 0.08 | 149.9 | 9.96 | 0.08 | 135.4 | 2362.3 | 2.12 |
| 3 | 0.09 | 137.1 | 0.11 | 354.1 | 23.52 | 0.15 | 22.4 | 8528.5 | 7.66 |
| 4 | 0.16 | 22.5 | 0.16 | 25.0 | 1.66 | 0.20 | 6.5 | 456.8 | 0.41 |
| 5 | 0.30 | 3.2 | 0.41 | 94.7 | 6.29 | 0.43 | 89.9 | 3070.0 | 2.76 |
| 6 | 0.47 | 83.8 | 0.52 | 213.5 | 14.18 | 0.57 | 138.4 | 10264.7 | 9.22 |
| 7 | 0.59 | 141.8 | 0.85 | 505.7 | 33.60 | 0.99 | 4.5 | 84211.4 | 75.60 |

## HPTLC Fingerprinting Profile of Karivepillai Chooranam

HPTLC fingerprint profile has been performed for the KVC . The HPTLC image for the ethonol extract of KVC under UV at 254 nm is presented in Fig 20. While, the HPTLC image for the ethonol extract of KVC under UV at 366 nm is shown in Fig 21.

The 3D densidometry chromatogram developed using 5 μl and 15 μl of test solution under 254 nm shows similer such peaks (Fig 22).

The HPTLC fingerprint using 5 μl of test solution under UV 254 nm shows nine major peak at the Rf values 0.09, 0.20, 0.27, 0.32, 0.45, 0.58, 0.77 and 0.85 with 15 μl of test solution under 254 nm eleven peaks were produced at the Rf values 0.09, 0.20, 0.28, 0.31, 0.44, 0.57, 0.66, 0.77, 0.85 and 0.94 (Fig 24 and Table 10). The highest peak a areas in the Rf 0.85 (5979 AU with 19.2%) was for 5 μl test solution while it was 0.94 (10546.3AU with 22.83 %) for 15 μl of test solution. The 3D densitometry chromatogram developed using 5 μl and 15 μl of test solution under 366 nm showed similer peaks (Fig 25). The HPTLC fingerprint pfofile of 5 μl test solution at 366 nm exhibited nine major peaks at Rf values 0.04, 0.14, 0.22, 0.26, 0.44, 0.73, 0.82 and 0.88; While the 15 μl of test.

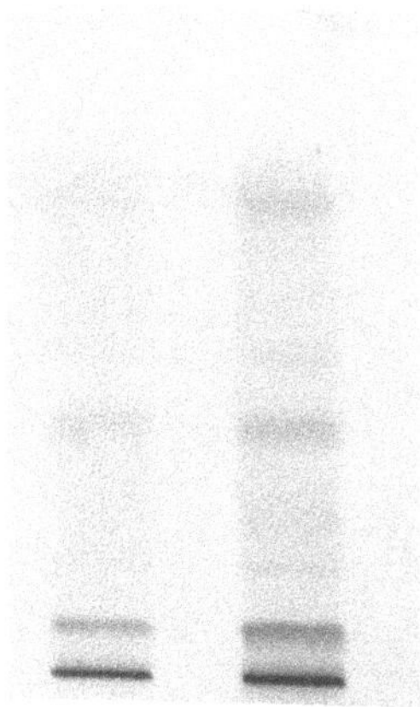

**5 μl 15 μl**
**Under UV at 254nm**

**Fig 20** HPTLC Fingerprint profile of the alcohol extract of KVC Under UV at 254nm

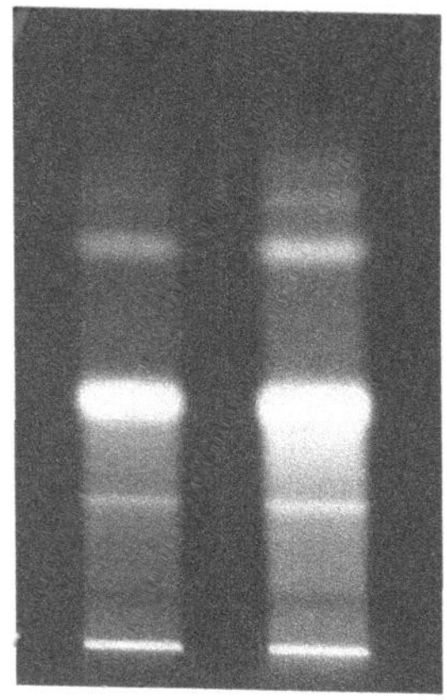

**5 μl 15 μl**
**Under UV at 366nm**

**Fig 21** HPTLC Fingerprint profile of the alcohol extract of Under UV at 366nm.

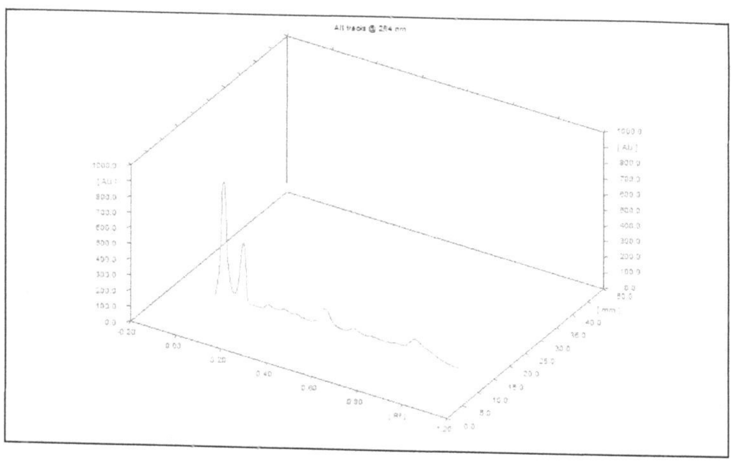

**Fig 22** The 3D densitometric chromatogram of 5 μl and 15 μl of alcohol extract of KVC 254 nm

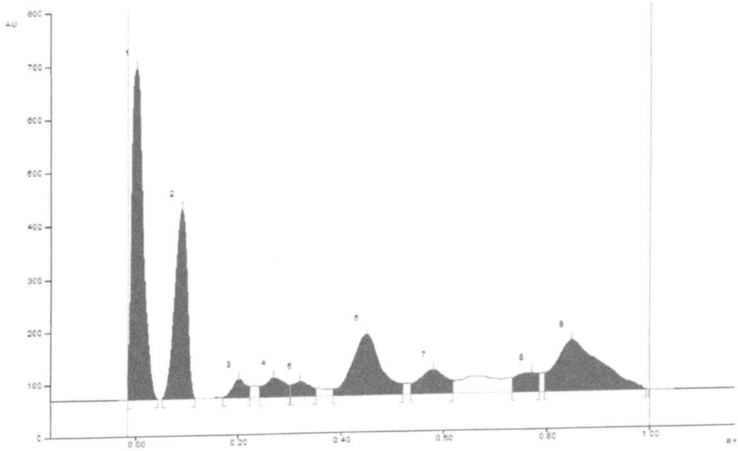

**Fig 23** HPTLC Fingerppint profile with peak displayfor 5µl of alcohol extract of KVC under UV at 254 nm

**Table 9** The Rf values for 5 µ1 of alcohol extract of KVC at 254nm

| Peak | Start Position | Start Height | Max Position | Max Height | Max % | End Position | End Height | Area | Area % |
|---|---|---|---|---|---|---|---|---|---|
| 1 | -0.01 Rf | 27.2 AU | 0.00 Rf | 623.5 AU | 45.33 % | 0.04 Rf | 0.6 AU | 9581.3 AU | 30.90 % |
| 2 | 0.05 Rf | 0.6 AU | 0.09 Rf | 359.2 AU | 26.11 % | 0.12 Rf | 0.8 AU | 5979.3 AU | 19.28 % |
| 3 | 0.17 Rf | 1.0 AU | 0.20 Rf | 34.9 AU | 2.54 % | 0.22 Rf | 21.4 AU | 652.3 AU | 2.10 % |
| 4 | 0.24 Rf | 20.5 AU | 0.27 Rf | 36.3 AU | 2.64 % | 0.30 Rf | 21.2 AU | 1040.9 AU | 3.36 % |
| 5 | 0.30 Rf | 21.4 AU | 0.32 Rf | 27.5 AU | 2.00 % | 0.35 Rf | 14.5 AU | 677.3 AU | 2.18 % |
| 6 | 0.38 Rf | 12.4 AU | 0.45 Rf | 116.1 AU | 8.44 % | 0.52 Rf | 19.6 AU | 4492.0 AU | 14.49 % |
| 7 | 0.54 Rf | 19.5 AU | 0.58 Rf | 45.3 AU | 3.29 % | 0.62 Rf | 24.4 AU | 1681.6 AU | 5.42 % |
| 8 | 0.74 Rf | 27.2 AU | 0.77 Rf | 36.0 AU | 2.62 % | 0.79 Rf | 34.2 AU | 1065.5 AU | 3.44 % |
| 9 | 0.80 Rf | 35.1 AU | 0.85 Rf | 96.7 AU | 7.03 % | 1.00 Rf | 1.2 AU | 5838.1 AU | 18.83 % |

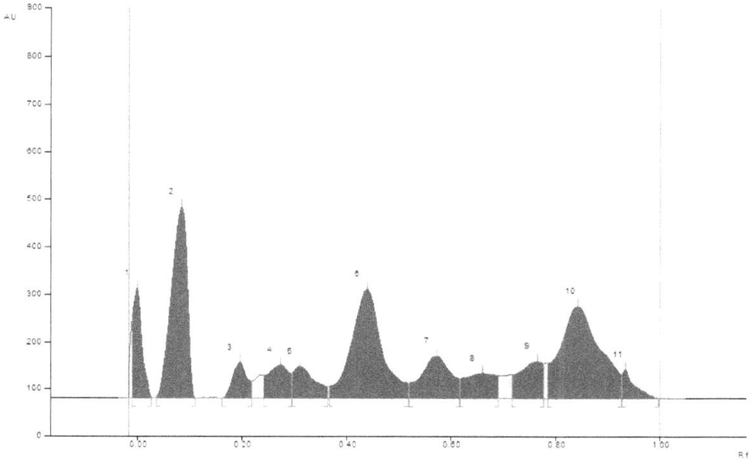

**Fig 24** 3D HPTLC Fingerpprint profile with peak displayfor 15µl of alcohol extract of KVC under UV at 254 nm

**Table 10** The Rf value for 15 µl of alcohol extract of KVC at 254nm

| Peak | Start Position | Start Height | Max Position | Max Height | Max % | End Position | End Height | Area | Area % |
|---|---|---|---|---|---|---|---|---|---|
| 1 | -0.01 Rf | 171.6 AU | 0.00 Rf | 233.7 AU | 14.89 % | 0.03 Rf | 2.3 AU | 2822.1 AU | 6.11 % |
| 2 | 0.04 Rf | 1.3 AU | 0.09 Rf | 402.9 AU | 25.67 % | 0.11 Rf | 0.1 AU | 8654.2 AU | 18.73 % |
| 3 | 0.16 Rf | 0.5 AU | 0.20 Rf | 77.7 AU | 4.95 % | 0.22 Rf | 36.1 AU | 1426.2 AU | 3.09 % |
| 4 | 0.24 Rf | 48.4 AU | 0.28 Rf | 72.2 AU | 4.60 % | 0.30 Rf | 52.6 AU | 1992.2 AU | 4.31 % |
| 5 | 0.30 Rf | 53.7 AU | 0.31 Rf | 68.2 AU | 4.34 % | 0.37 Rf | 24.8 AU | 1935.3 AU | 4.19 % |
| 6 | 0.37 Rf | 25.3 AU | 0.44 Rf | 231.4 AU | 14.74 % | 0.52 Rf | 32.2 AU | 9486.3 AU | 20.53 % |
| 7 | 0.52 Rf | 32.4 AU | 0.57 Rf | 91.5 AU | 5.83 % | 0.62 Rf | 42.4 AU | 3612.3 AU | 7.82 % |
| 8 | 0.62 Rf | 42.5 AU | 0.66 Rf | 53.7 AU | 3.42 % | 0.69 Rf | 48.9 AU | 2169.9 AU | 4.70 % |
| 9 | 0.72 Rf | 50.1 AU | 0.77 Rf | 79.9 AU | 5.09 % | 0.78 Rf | 77.2 AU | 2573.8 AU | 5.57 % |
| 10 | 0.79 Rf | 76.4 AU | 0.85 Rf | 195.5 AU | 12.46 % | 0.93 Rf | 52.9 AU | 10546.3 AU | 22.83 % |
| 11 | 0.93 Rf | 54.3 AU | 0.94 Rf | 63.1 AU | 4.02 % | 1.00 Rf | 0.4 AU | 977.7 AU | 2.12 % |

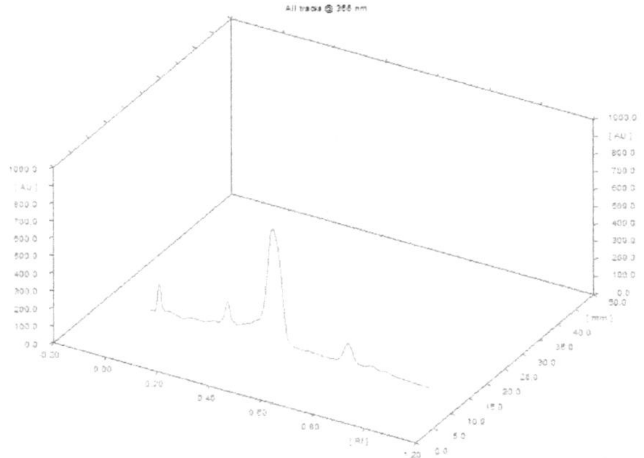

**Fig 25** The 3D densidometric chromatogram of 5 µl and 15 µl of alchol extract of KVC at 360 nm

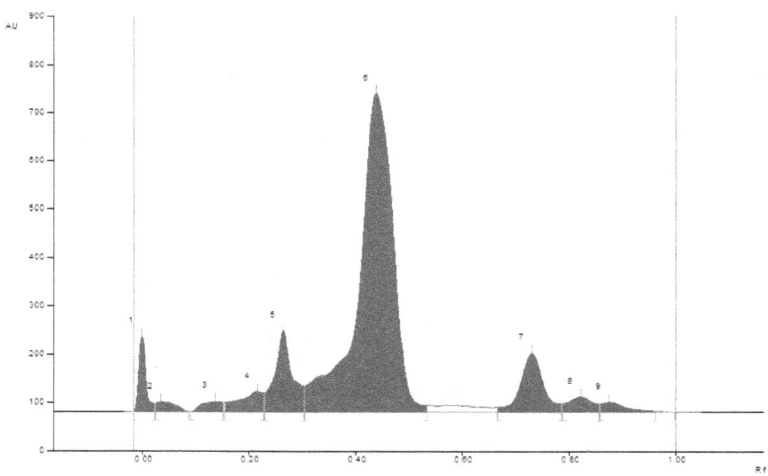


**Fig 26** HPTLC fingerprinting profile with peak display for 5µl of alcohol extract of KVC at 366 nm

**Table 11** The Rf values for 5 μl of alcohol extract of KVC at 360nm

| Peak | Start Position | Start Height | Max Position | Max Height | Max % | End Position | End Height | Area | Area % |
|---|---|---|---|---|---|---|---|---|---|
| 1 | -0.01 Rf | 1.2 AU | 0.00 Rf | 156.2 AU | 12.58 % | 0.03 Rf | 17.4 AU | 1544.4 AU | 3.60 % |
| 2 | 0.03 Rf | 17.6 AU | 0.04 Rf | 20.4 AU | 1.64 % | 0.09 Rf | 0.1 AU | 517.3 AU | 1.21 % |
| 3 | 0.09 Rf | 0.1 AU | 0.14 Rf | 21.9 AU | 1.77 % | 0.15 Rf | 20.0 AU | 593.4 AU | 1.38 % |
| 4 | 0.16 Rf | 19.9 AU | 0.22 Rf | 42.5 AU | 3.42 % | 0.23 Rf | 39.5 AU | 1330.5 AU | 3.10 % |
| 5 | 0.23 Rf | 39.9 AU | 0.26 Rf | 168.3 AU | 13.55 % | 0.31 Rf | 54.4 AU | 3958.4 AU | 9.23 % |
| 6 | 0.31 Rf | 54.6 AU | 0.44 Rf | 658.8 AU | 53.06 % | 0.54 Rf | 13.1 AU | 29619.1 AU | 69.07 % |
| 7 | 0.67 Rf | 9.8 AU | 0.73 Rf | 121.8 AU | 9.81 % | 0.79 Rf | 17.3 AU | 3624.4 AU | 8.45 % |
| 8 | 0.79 Rf | 17.5 AU | 0.82 Rf | 31.5 AU | 2.54 % | 0.86 Rf | 16.7 AU | 1025.5 AU | 2.39 % |
| 9 | 0.86 Rf | 16.8 AU | 0.88 Rf | 20.3 AU | 1.64 % | 0.96 Rf | 2.1 AU | 667.3 AU | 1.56 % |

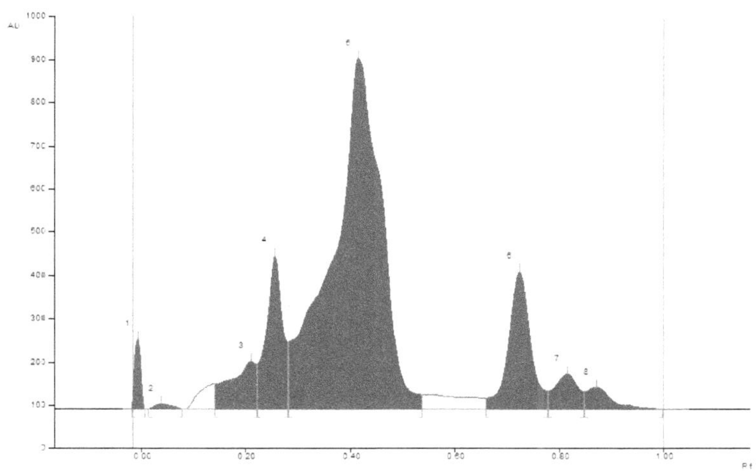

**Fig 27** HPTLC fingerprinting profile with peak display for15μl of alcohol extract of KVC at575 nm

**Table 12** The Rf values for 15 μl of alcohol extract of KVC

| Peak | Start Position | Start Height | Max Position | Max Height | Max % | End Position | End Height | Area | Area % |
|---|---|---|---|---|---|---|---|---|---|
| 1 | -0.02 Rf | 0.0 AU | -0.00 Rf | 160.7 AU | 8.45 % | 0.01 Rf | 0.4 AU | 1373.5 AU | 1.73 % |
| 2 | 0.01 Rf | 0.8 AU | 0.04 Rf | 11.7 AU | 0.62 % | 0.08 Rf | 0.2 AU | 260.3 AU | 0.33 % |
| 3 | 0.14 Rf | 57.9 AU | 0.21 Rf | 110.2 AU | 5.80 % | 0.22 Rf | 04.2 AU | 3886.2 AU | 4.88 % |
| 4 | 0.22 Rf | 104.6 AU | 0.26 Rf | 353.1 AU | 18.57 % | 0.28 Rf | 56.0 AU | 7750.2 AU | 9.74 % |
| 5 | 0.28 Rf | 156.1 AU | 0.42 Rf | 814.0 AU | 42.81 % | 0.54 Rf | 33.8 AU | 52624.3 AU | 66.12 % |
| 6 | 0.66 Rf | 26.0 AU | 0.73 Rf | 318.1 AU | 16.73 % | 0.78 Rf | 42.8 AU | 9434.9 AU | 11.85 % |
| 7 | 0.78 Rf | 42.9 AU | 0.82 Rf | 82.4 AU | 4.33 % | 0.85 Rf | 41.1 AU | 2513.6 AU | 3.16 % |
| 8 | 0.85 Rf | 41.1 AU | 0.87 Rf | 50.9 AU | 2.68 % | 1.00 Rf | 0.0 AU | 1744.6 AU | 2.19 % |

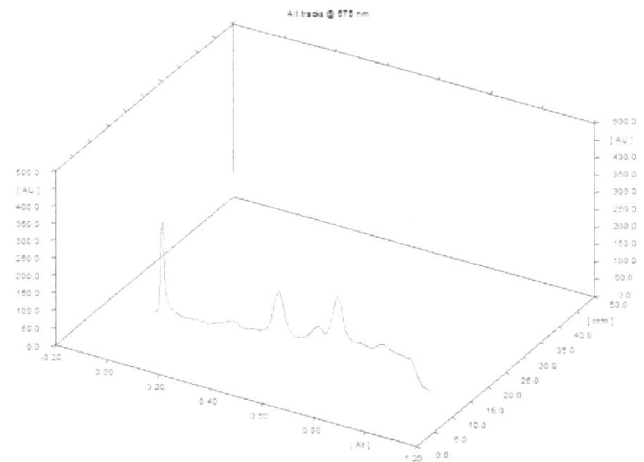


**Fig 27** The 3D densitometric chromatogram of 5 µl and 15 µl of alcohol extract of KVC at 575 nm after derivatisation

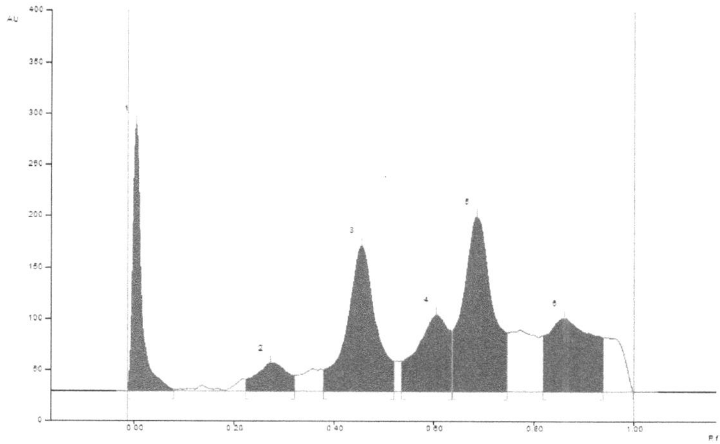

**Fig 28** HPTLC fingerprinting profile with peak display for 5µl of alcohol extract of KVC at 575 nm

**Table 13** The Rf value for 5 µl of alcohol extract of KVC at 575 nm

| Peak | Start Position | Start Height | Max Position | Max Height | Max % | End Position | End Height | Area | Area % |
|---|---|---|---|---|---|---|---|---|---|
| 1 | -0.01 Rf | 1.7 AU | 0.00 Rf | 260.4 AU | 34.87 % | 0.08 Rf | 1.5 AU | 3130.8 AU | 12.70 % |
| 2 | 0.22 Rf | 11.7 AU | 0.28 Rf | 27.6 AU | 3.69 % | 0.32 Rf | 15.4 AU | 1212.3 AU | 4.92 % |
| 3 | 0.38 Rf | 21.2 AU | 0.46 Rf | 142.3 AU | 19.05 % | 0.52 Rf | 29.3 AU | 5628.4 AU | 22.84 % |
| 4 | 0.54 Rf | 29.4 AU | 0.61 Rf | 74.3 AU | 9.96 % | 0.64 Rf | 59.0 AU | 3265.5 AU | 13.25 % |
| 5 | 0.64 Rf | 59.4 AU | 0.69 Rf | 170.4 AU | 22.82 % | 0.75 Rf | 57.6 AU | 6946.3 AU | 28.18 % |
| 6 | 0.82 Rf | 54.8 AU | 0.86 Rf | 71.8 AU | 9.62 % | 0.94 Rf | 52.7 AU | 4463.4 AU | 18.11 % |

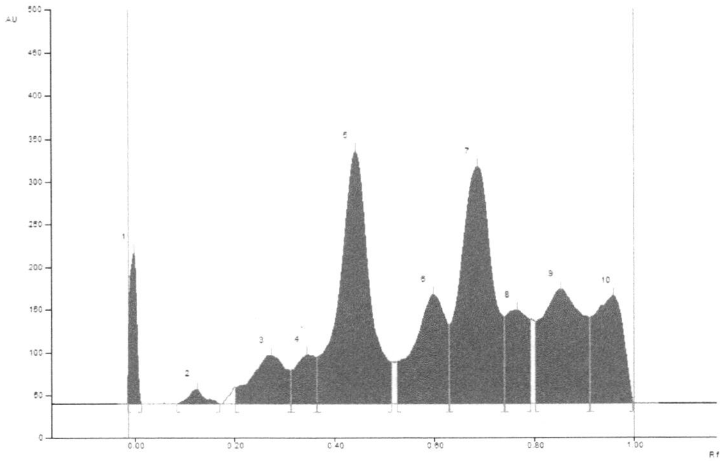

**Fig 29** HPTLC fingerprinting profile with peak display for 15μl of alcohol extract of KVC at 575 nm

**Tabe 14** The Rf value for 15 μl of alcohol extract of KVC at 575 nm

| Peak | Start Position | Start Height | Max Position | Max Height | Max % | End Position | End Height | Area | Area % |
|---|---|---|---|---|---|---|---|---|---|
| 1 | -0.01 Rf | 0.0 AU | 0.00 Rf | 178.2 AU | 12.93 % | 0.01 Rf | 0.0 AU | 1737.9 AU | 3.33 % |
| 2 | 0.09 Rf | 0.0 AU | 0.13 Rf | 17.1 AU | 1.24 % | 0.17 Rf | 0.3 AU | 373.4 AU | 0.72 % |
| 3 | 0.20 Rf | 19.2 AU | 0.28 Rf | 56.9 AU | 4.13 % | 0.31 Rf | 39.4 AU | 2697.6 AU | 5.17 % |
| 4 | 0.31 Rf | 39.4 AU | 0.34 Rf | 57.5 AU | 4.17 % | 0.37 Rf | 54.0 AU | 1586.2 AU | 3.04 % |
| 5 | 0.37 Rf | 54.4 AU | 0.44 Rf | 295.4 AU | 21.43 % | 0.51 Rf | 48.9 AU | 12313.2 AU | 23.58 % |
| 6 | 0.53 Rf | 49.2 AU | 0.60 Rf | 127.5 AU | 9.25 % | 0.63 Rf | 92.3 AU | 5663.7 AU | 10.85 % |
| 7 | 0.63 Rf | 92.5 AU | 0.69 Rf | 277.5 AU | 20.13 % | 0.74 Rf | 01.2 AU | 12083.7 AU | 23.14 % |
| 8 | 0.74 Rf | 101.5 AU | 0.77 Rf | 109.2 AU | 7.92 % | 0.79 Rf | 98.3 AU | 3257.8 AU | 6.24 % |
| 9 | 0.80 Rf | 95.3 AU | 0.86 Rf | 133.7 AU | 9.70 % | 0.91 Rf | 00.4 AU | 7588.8 AU | 14.53 % |
| 10 | 0.92 Rf | 100.6 AU | 0.96 Rf | 125.4 AU | 9.10 % | 1.00 Rf | 5.1 AU | 4909.3 AU | 9.40 % |

Solution at 366nm shows seven peaks at Rf values 0.04, 0.21, 0.26, 0.42, 0.73, 0.82, and 0.87 (Fig 27 and Table 12) . The highest peak area found at the Rf value with maximum peak areas for 5μl and 15μl test solution are 29619.1AU (69.07%) at the Rf value of 0.44 and 52624.3AU(66.12%) at the Rf values 0.42 respectively.The 3D Densitometry chromatogram developed using 5µl and 15µl of test solution under 575 nm afterderivatization using vanillin –sulphuric acid reagent shows similar patterns of peaks (Fig 27). HPTLC fingerprinting profile of 5µl test solution at 575nm show 6 major peaks at Rf values 0.00, 0.28, 0.46, 0.61, 0.69, 0.86 and (Fig 28 and Table 13) while that of 15 µl of test solution shows eight peaks at Rf values19.2, 39.4, 54.4, 49.2, 92.5, 101.5, 95.3, 100.6 (Fig 29 and Table 13). The highest peak area found at the Rf value with maximum Peak Areas for 5µl and 15µl test solution are 6946.3AU(28.18%) at the Rf 0.69 and 12313.2AU (23.58%) at the Rf 0.44 respectively.

## 5.2 Antioxidant Activity Studies

### Results ABTS, DPPH and Nitric Oxide (NO) Radical Assay

A gradual increase in the antioxidant activity of KVC results in the corresponding inhibition of the ABTS radical. The ABTS Assay displayed that KVC of 6.25, 12.5, 25.50 and 100 g/ml concentration and the corresponding percentage of inhibition was, *viz.*, 47.86 ± 2 ± 43, 74.06 ± 2.01, 96.54 ± 0.50, and 98.27 ± 0.75 respectively (Table 14, Fig 30). IC 50 was found to be at 13.51 ± 1.24

**Table 14** The Antioxidant Activity Of KVC For ABTS Radical Analysis

| S.No | Concentration (ʃg/ml) | % Inhibition | IC50 (µg/ml) |
|---|---|---|---|
| 1 | 100 | 98.27 ±0.75 | 13.51 ± 1.24 |
| 2 | 50 | 96.54 ±0.50 | |
| 3 | 25 | 74.06 ± 2.01 | |
| 4 | 12.5 | 47.86 ± 2.43 | |
| 5 | 6.25 | 43.24 ±3.15 | |
| 6 | IC 50 | 13.51 ±1.24 | |

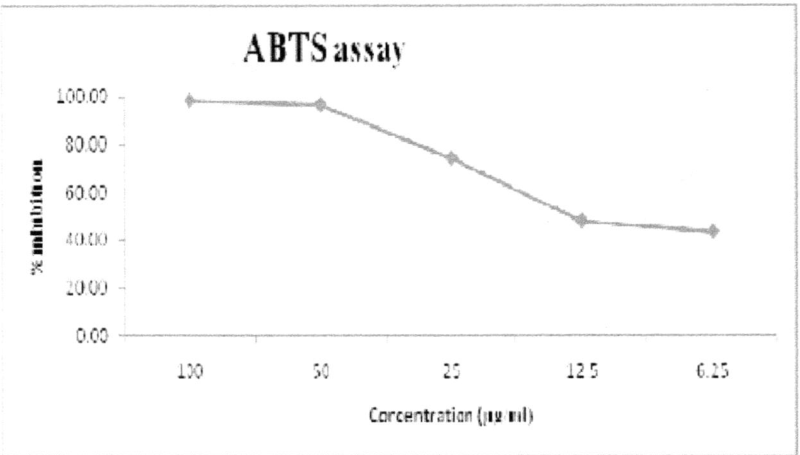


**Fig 30** Graphical Representation Of ABTS Inhibitory Activity Of KVC

**Table 15** The antioxidant activity of KVC for DPPH radical.

±

| S. No | Concentration (⌠g/ml) | % Inhibition | IC50 (µg/ml) |
|---|---|---|---|
| 1 | 1000 | 89.02±0.37 | 240.25±0.36 |
| 2 | 500 | 86.01±0.76 | |
| 3 | 250 | 51.93±0.99 | |
| 4 | 125 | 27.28±0.83 | |
| 5 | 62.5 | 16.14±0.52 | |
| 6 | IC 50 | 240.25±0.36 | |

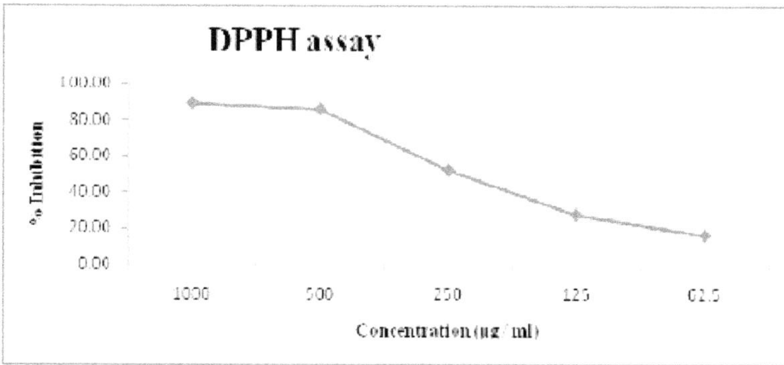


**Fig 31** Graphical representation of DPPH inhibitory activity for kariveppillai choornam

Antioxidant activity of the test substance for DPPH radicalassay showed a progressive inhibition of DPPH radicles in the increasing concerntration of KVC . the percentage of inhibition for 62.5,125,250,500 and 1000 mg/ml concerntrationof KVC was 16.14±0.52,27.28±0.83,51.93±0.99,86.01±0.76,89. And 02±0.37 respectively. The IC 50 obtained was 240.25 ± 0.36. (Table 15 and Fig 31)

**Table 16** The antioxidant activity of KVC for Nitric oxide radical

| S.No | Concentration (⌠g/ml) | % Inhibition | IC50 (µg/ml) |
|---|---|---|---|
| 1 | 1000 | 52.59±0.34 | 865.03±0.88 |
| 2 | 500 | 43..03±0.39 | |
| 3 | 250 | 34.32±1.46 | |
| 4 | 125 | 13.75±1.21 | |
| 5 | 62.5 | 3.64±2.35 | |
| 6 | IC 50 | 865.03±0.88 | |

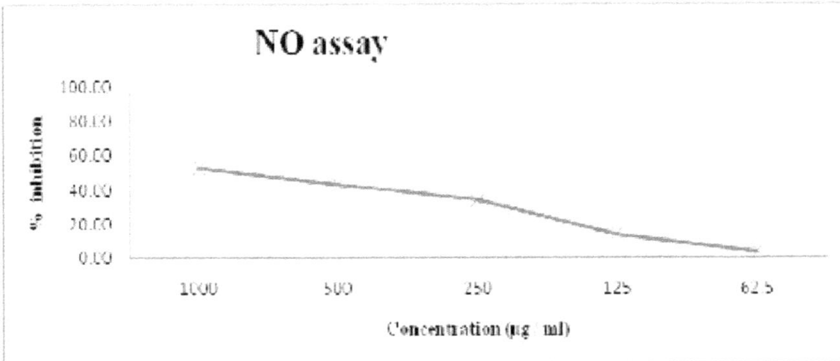


**Fig 32** Graphical representation of nitricoxide radical inhibitory activity for the KVC

Table 16 Fig 32 exhibition Antioxidant activity KVC for NO radicals with the increacing concerntrations of KVC., 62.5,125,250,500 and 1000 mg/ml was found with the % inhibition of 3.64 ± 2.35, 13.75 ± 1.21, 34.32 ± 1.46, 43.03±0.39, and 52.59 ± 0.34 respectively. The IC 50 was found to be 865.03 ± 0.88. (Table 16, Fig 32)

The gradual concentration Anti-oxidant activity of test substance for ABTS radicals showed that increase in concerntration has inhibition of the ABTS radicals. The IC 50 was found to be 13.51± 1.24. Okaka and Okaka (2001) had also reported similer results from their studies

The antioxidant activity of test substance for DPPH radical with increase in the effective concentration resulted in gradual effective inhibition of DPPH radical. IC 50 obtained was 240.25 ± 0.36. This was in confirmity with Jao and Ko (2002) who had explined DPPH radical scavengive activity for the natural food juice.

Anti-oxidant activity of test substance for NO radical showed that gradual increase in the concentration of the drug resulted in gradual inhibition of NO radical. IC 50 was found to be 865.03 = 0.88. These results are in accordance with those of Bandyopadhyay and Das (1999), and Serdan and Ahmet (2007).

So,The antioxidant activity of karivepillai choornam (KVC) is assessed in the method of ABTS, DPPH and NO2,found very good inhibition of high to low level concentration. Similer such results were shown by Uday (1999) in *Muraya Koenigii.*

## 5.3 Antimicrobial And Antiadipogenesis Studies

### 5.3 Results Of Antibacterial Studies

**Antibacterial Activity**

The results of the microbiological analysis for microbial contamination of the drug KVC are given in Table 18. The total viable aerobic bacterial counts on Nutrient agar plate was 21 x $10^2$ CFU / g and the fungal count on SDA agar plates was 2x$10^1$ CFU/ g. This results were found to comply with the specification limit for total bacterial count i.e. NMT $1\times 10^5$ CFU/ml and total fungal count, i.e., NMT $1\times10^3$ CFU/ml as per the Frotoccl for testing Ayurveda, Siddha and Unani medicines (Table 18).

The analytical screening of sample is shown in Table 19. The KVC istested for its contamination if any with the human pathogens like *Escherichia coli*, *Salmonella* sp., *Pseudomonas aeruginosa* and *Staphylococcus aureus.* Microbial contamination usually occurs because of improper drying or storage of the plant material which eventually results in degradation of the plant constituents. Microbial contamination can also render plant material toxic, either by transforming the chemicals in the plant material or through the production of toxic compounds by the microbes. Therefore, The microbial quality tests are nessary for the plant materials, intermediates and finished products hence. During the quality analysis, precautions must be taken to ensure that conditions are not adversely affected any by microorganisms.

Thus, the present study proves that KVC is free from microbial contamination and also highlighted the safety of the same. The information obtained from microbial screening tests will be useful in finding out the quality of the drug. The good antibacterial activity of herbal medicines indicate that the antimicrobial compounds present in herbal medicines are possibly controlling the microbial activity. Herbal medicines, in genaral showe varying degrees of *in vitro* antibacterial activity against test bacteria.

**Table 18** The Results Of Bacterial Contamination Test

| S.No. | Test Particulars | Colony Counts (CFU/ g) | Limits Value (CFU/g) |
|---|---|---|---|
| 1. | Total Viable Aerobic Bacterial Count | $20 \times 10^2$ | $1 \times 10^5$ |
| 2. | Total Viable Fungal Count | $2 \times 10^1$ | $1 \times 10^3$ |

**Table 19** Results Of Specific Pathogens Test

| S.No. | Test for Specified Pathogens | Colony Counts (CFU/ g) | Limits Value (CFU/g) |
|---|---|---|---|
| 1. | *Salmonella* sp. | No growth | - |
| 2. | *Staphylococcus aureus* | No growth | - |
| 3. | *Escherichia coli* | No growth | - |
| 4. | *Pseudomonas aeruginosa* | No growth | - |

*Escherichia coli, Staphylococcus aureus,* and *Pseudomonas aeruginosa* were found to be more sensitive to the KVC compared to the standard drug gentamycin (Broad spectrum) (Table 20, Figure 33). The Zone of inhibition (mm) shown by control (Gentamycin) were 26 mm, 23mm, 23mm, 22mm and 21mm and test drug KVC showed 23mm, 20mm, 21mm, 18mm and 19mm respectively (Table 20). The aqueous extract of KVC showed significant zone of inhibition when compared to the standard antibiotic Gentamycin and no zone of inhibition was observed in negative control.The highest zone of inhibition was found in Escheria coli (23mm) and the least inhibition was against *Pseudomonas aeruginosa* (18mm). The fact that the extracts were active agains sevaral bacteria indicate the broad spectrum of activity by KVC. Hence the herbal drug, KVC exhibited broad spectrum activity against bacterial pathogens at 100mg / ml concentration of the drug.

The phytochemical screening of KVC showed the presence of phenol, tannins and flavonods, Phytochemicals have inhibited the microorganism by impairing the enzymes involved in energy production, interfering the integrity of cell membrane and structural component synthesis, The growth of bacteria have been inhibited due to the presence of phenolic compounds (Nithya *et al*, 2014). It is accomplished from this study that the results lead to the establishment of several important compounds that have to be used to formulate new, different and more potent antimicrobial drugs of natural origin. However, further detile studies on the biologically active compounds and their evaluation the efficiency against pathogenic microorganisms of various human diseases are required for the new drug discovery and formulation

**Table 20** Antibacterial Activities of Drug by Agar Well Diffusion Method

| S.No. | Test Pathogens | Result | Zone of Inhibition (mm) at 30µl | |
|---|---|---|---|---|
| | | | Positive Control (Gentamycin) | Size of Inhibition |
| 1. | *Escherichia coli* | Sensitive | 26 mm | 23 mm |
| 2 | *Staphylococcus aureus* | Sensitive | 23 mm | 21 mm |
| 3 | *Pseudomonas aeruginosa* | Sensitive | 22 mm | 18 mm |

***A. Escherichia coli***

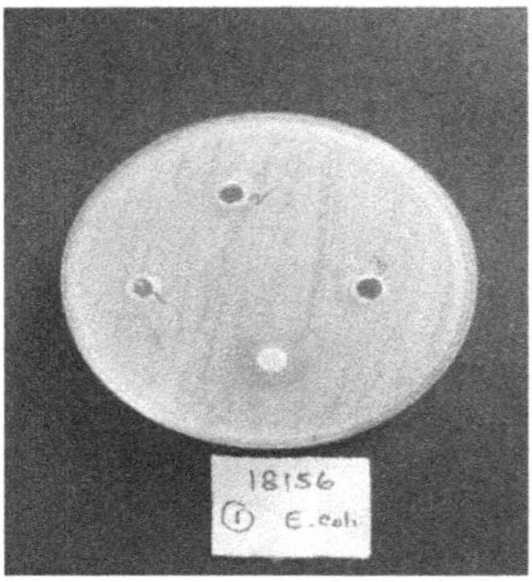


***B. Staphylococcus aureus***

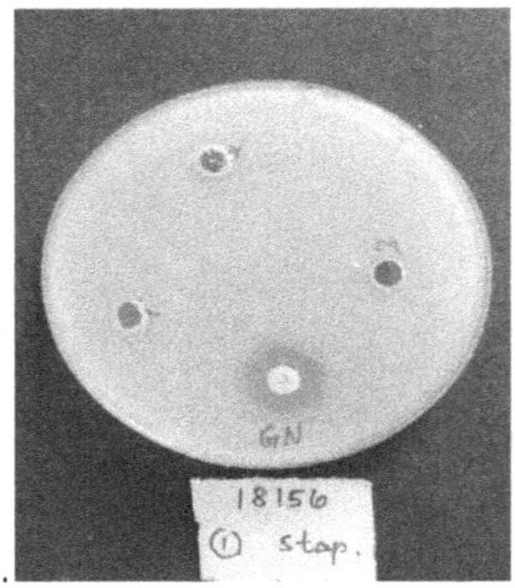


***C. Pseudomonas aeruginosa***

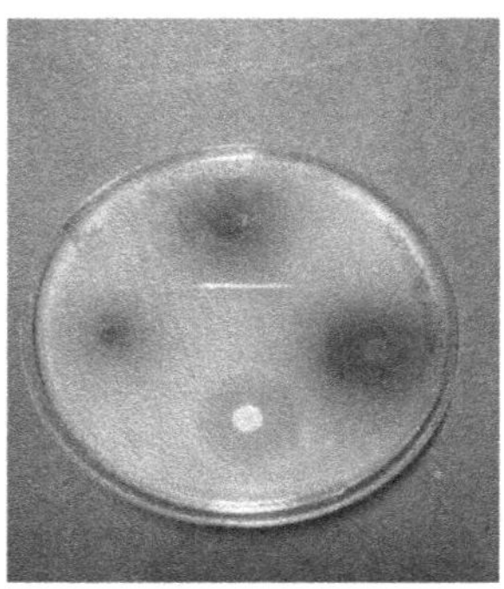

**Fig 33** The zone of inhibition by the KVC extract

### 5.3b Antifungal Activity Dicussion

The Potato Dextrose Agar medium (HiMedia) plate was used in this study, The KVC were tested against two fungi, The antifungal activity was carried out by Disc Diffusion Plate Method (Mackie and Cartney,1989; Pelczar and Cham, 2005). The KVC antifungals potential of KVC against selected pathogens were compared with the standared antifungal drug (Clotrimazole). Diameter of Zone of inhibition for 250, 500 and 1000 μg/ml of KVC were measured using Zone Reader and are given in Table 21 and 22. At the end of the stucy it is found that Aspergillus niger and Canadia albicans showed the values of 32,10,12,14 and 41,11,13 respectively (Fig 34 and 35). In *Candia albicans* there was no zone of inhibition in the dose of 250μg/ml.

The qualitative phytochemical screening of KVC showed the presence of phenolic compunds, glycosides, amino acids and are presence of constituents like a fluvanoids, tannins and triterpenoids in the KVC extracts which are responsible for the antimicrobial activity (Bose and Mondal 2007).

**Table 21** Antifungal activity of the aqueous extract of KVC against *Aspergillus niger*

| Organism | Concentration of KVC (μg/ml) | Zone of inhibition (mm) |
|---|---|---|
| *Aspergillus niger* | Clotrimazole | 32 |
| | 250 | 10 |
| | 500 | 12 |
| | 1000 | 14 |

**Table 22** Antifungal activity of the aqueous extract of KVC against *Candida albicans*

| **Organism** | **Concentration of KVC (µg/mL)** | **Zone of inhibition (mm)** |
|---|---|---|
| ***Candida albicans*** | Clotrimazole | 41 |
| | 250 | Nil |
| | 500 | 11 |
| | 1000 | 13 |

***Average of 3 replicates**

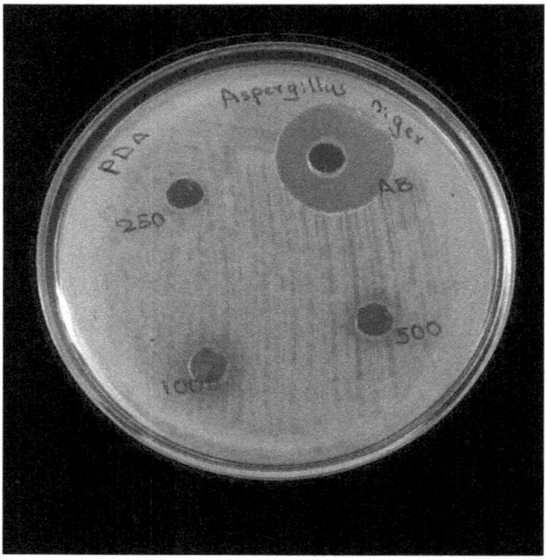


**Fig 34** The Zone Of Inhibition In *Aspergillus niger* (ATCC 16404)

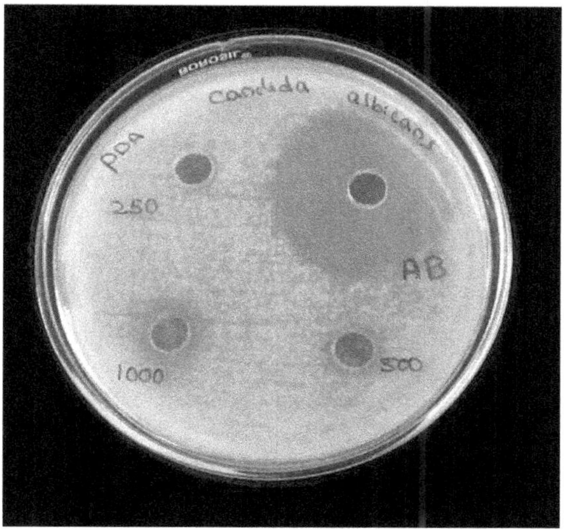


**Fig 35** The zone of Inhibition in *Candida albicans* (ATCC 10234)

## 5.3 c Results of Hypolipidemic Activity

## Antiadipogenesis Studies

The concentration level of 100 μg/ml and 200 μg/ml, of KVC and the lipogenic inhibition for the test soultion concentration of 100 and 200 μg/ml were at 15% and 25% respectively (Fig 37). The N1, N2 and N3 average percentage inhibition is 16.2±4.97, 17.1±2.63, 16.6 and 24.4±2.21, 25.8±1.57 and 25.1±1 respectivly. (Table 23)

**Table 23** *In vitro* anti-adipogenisis activity of KVC

| Test Concentration (µg/ml) | Percentage Inhibition Over Control (AVG±SD) | | |
|---|---|---|---|
| | N1 | N2 | N3 |
| 200 | 24.4±2.21 | 25.8±1.57 | 25.1±1 |
| 100 | 16.2±4.97 | 17.1±2.63 | 16.6 |

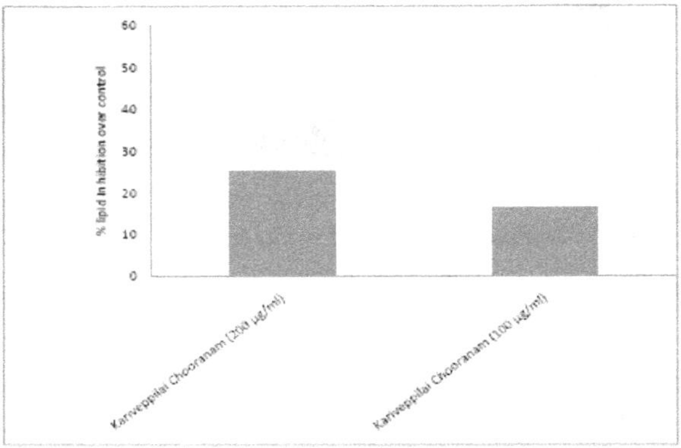


**Fig 31** Invitro anti-adipogenesis effect of KVC

As per the Table 24 Figure 38 at a KVC concentration of 100 µg/ml and 200 µg/ml and corresponding fraction of free glycerol released were found to be 130% and 120% respectively. (Fig 38) The level of released triglyceride in cell supernatant is 134. 53± 1.38 and 119 .82 ±0.90 respectively for 100 and 200 µg/ml concerntration of KVC (Table 24).

**Table 24** The level of released Triglyceride in cell supernatant

| S.No | Test Conc. (µg/ml) | Triglyceride mg/dl (% control) |
|---|---|---|
| 1 | 200 | 119.82±0.90 |
| 2 | 100 | 134.53±1.38 |

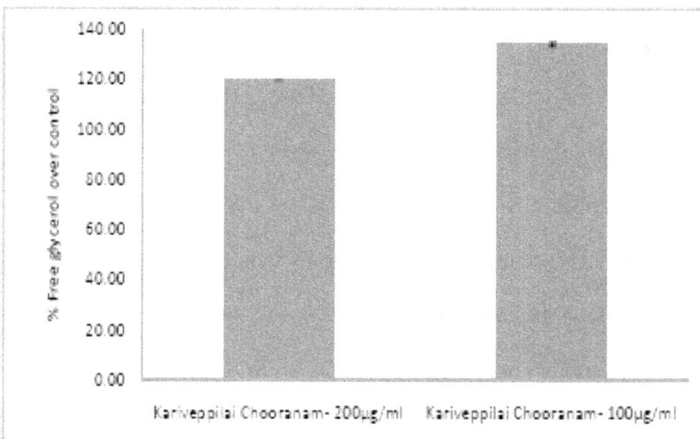


**Fig 32** The percentage level of released Triglyceride in cell supernatant

## *In vivo* Hypolipidemic Activity

The Wister albino rats were made to fast 12 hours, before the the induction of hyperlipidemia.There after Group IV &V group of animals were treated with KVC 100 and 200mg/kg/bw for 15 to 30 days. Group I & II are considered Normal and as Cholesterol control respectivly. Group III (standard control group) rats were fed Atorvastatin 1mg/kg/bw for 15 to 30 days ( Vijaya and Ramachandran, 2009).At the end of the study, a lipid profile of treatment control group (4 & 5) were observed; dose 100 to 200mg/kg/bw treated animals were the most responsible in lowering the Cholesterol, Triglycerides, HDL, LDL, VLDL, AI and LDL / HDL ratio. The lipid profile results for 100 mg of KVC were 94.50±3.22, 118.40±3.15, 18.20±0.95, 25.28±18.20±0.94, 4.30±1.30 and 1.38. Where as for 200mg 84.80±2.95, 99.35±3.05, 21.45±1.20, 22.05±1.48, 22.40±1.55, 3.15±0.90 and 1.02 were obtained for cholesterol, triglycerides, HDL, LDL, VLDL, AI and LDL / HDL respectively. Serum of hyperlipidemic rats showed significantly increased levels of cholesterol, triglycerides, LDL - C and low HDL – C, when compared with normal rats. In rats treated with both doses of herbal Siddha formulation of KVC and Atorvastatin, there was a significant decrease in the cholesterol, TGs, LDL – C, and VLDL increases HDL – C, when compared with cholesterol control rats.

The findings from *In vivo* study revealed that the mean effective doses or leathal dose of KVC had been investigated on dose 100-200 mg/ kg/ BW with no mortality being recorded or any manifestation of toxicity observed after the period of 30 days.

**Table 25** The Results of lipid profile of 5 groups test organisms after KVC treatment

| Groups | Total Cholesterol (Mg/Dl) | Triglycerides (Mg/Dl) | HDL (Mg/Dl) | LDL (Mg/Dl) | VLDL (Mg/Dl) | AI | LDL/HDL |
|---|---|---|---|---|---|---|---|
| Normal Control | 55.80 ± 2.40 | 68.35± 2.58 | 30.68 ± 1.30 | 15.26 ± 0.65 | 34.86 ± 2.20 | 0.49 ± 0.18 | 0.49 ± |
| Cholesterol Control | 122.15 ± 4.90$^{**(a)}$ | 172.50 ± 4.70$^{**(a)}$ | 10.95 ± 0.48$^{**(a)}$ | 31.68 ± 1.75$^{**(a)}$ | 16.30 ± 0.70$^{**(a)}$ | 8.48 ± 1.60$^{**(a)}$ | 2.89$^{**(a)}$ |
| Standard Control | 78.40± 2.84$^{**(b)}$ | 88.15± 2.85$^{**(b)}$ | 23.22 ± 1.32$^{**(b)}$ | 20.15 ± 1.22$^{**(b)}$ | 24.72 ± 1.70$^{**(b)}$ | 2.24 ± 0.76$^{**(b)}$ | 0.86$^{**(b)}$ |
| Treatment control (100 mg) | 94.50 ± 3.22$^{*(b)}$ | 118.40 ± 3.15$^{**(b)}$ | 18.20± 0.95$^{**(b)}$ | 25.28 ± 1.63$^{**(b)}$ | 18.20 ± 0.94$^{**(b)}$ | 4.30 ± 1.30$^{**(b)}$ | 1.38$^{**(b)}$ |
| Treatment control (200 mg) | 84.80 ± 2.95$^{**(b)}$ | 99.35± 3.05$^{**(b)}$ | 21.45 ± 1.20$^{**(b)}$ | 22.05± 1.48$^{**(b)}$ | 22.40 ± 1.55$^{**(b)}$ | 3.15 ± 0.90$^{**(b)}$ | 1.02$^{**(b)}$ |

- Values are expressed as Mean ± SEM.
- Values were found out by using ONE WAY ANOVA followed by Newman Keul's multiple range tests.

** (a) and ** (b) values significantly different from normal control at P< 0.01 and hyperlidemic control at P< 0.01 respectively.

**Atherogenic Index - LDL – C / HDL- C Ratio**

The Atherogenic Index and LDL – C / HDL – C ratio in control and treated rats are presented in Table 25. It is evident from these results that the cholesterol induction significantly affects the cardio vascular risk markers.

Indeed, AI got statistically increased (90%) in cholesterol control group compared to the values found in their normal control group.

There were also significant increase of LDL – C / HDL – C ratio in cholesterol control group compared to normal control group.

Promising results in lowering of AI by herbal Siddha formulation of KVC was found in Table 25. The herbal Siddha formulation of KVC showed an improvement of the cardio vascular risk level by decrease of AI in the treated group by more than 73% and 63% ($p < 0.01$), when compared to the cholesterol control group.

The ratio of LDL – C to HDL – C is also a protective indicator of cardio vascular disease incidence. The cholesterol induction produced a significant increase of this marker. In contrast, elevated ratio in treated group and Atorvastatin group returned to basal value when the data were compared with those data in the same period found for the cholesterol rats. (Table 25).

The groups IV and group V were organisms treated with KVC of different rats doses , where as group III rats were, treated with modern dry group II rats were cholesterol induced rats, and group I rats were normal saline fed rats. Fig 39 shows the effect of KVC even at lower dose (100 mg/ kg body weight) yielded results similar to those of Atorvastation treated rats. Similar results were obtained for the total triglycerides (Fig 40), HDL (Fig 41), LDL (Fig 42), VLDL (Fig 43), AI (Fig 44) and LDL/HDL (Fig 45).

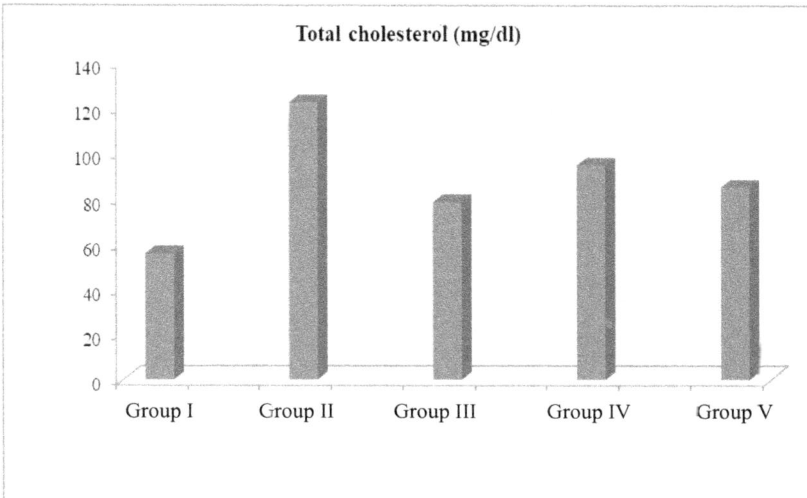


**Fig 39** Total cholesterol Variation among the 5 groups of test organisms after KVC adminstation

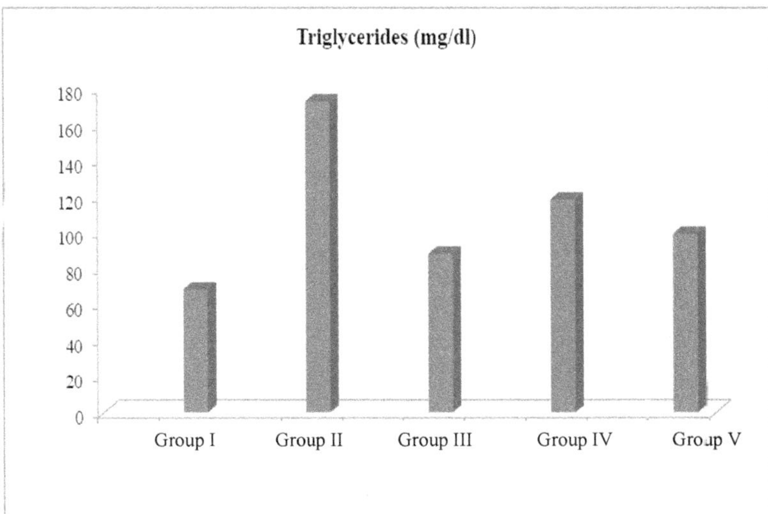


**Fig 40** Total Triglycerides Variation among the 5 groups of ten organisms after KVC treatment

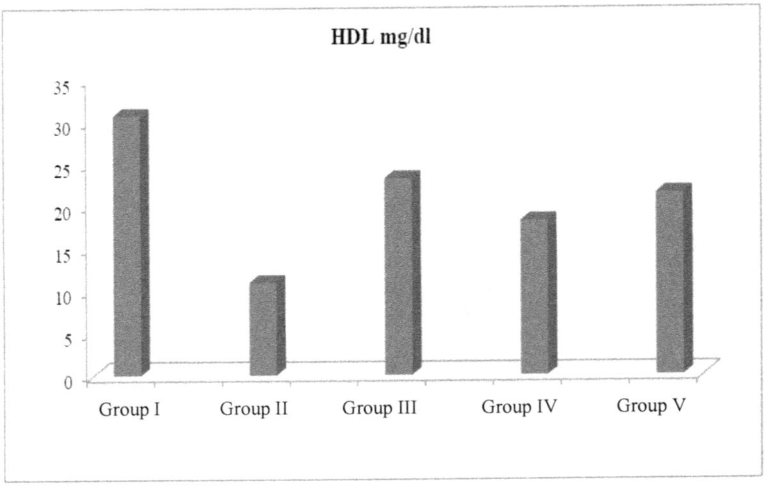


**Fig 41** Results of HDL Variation

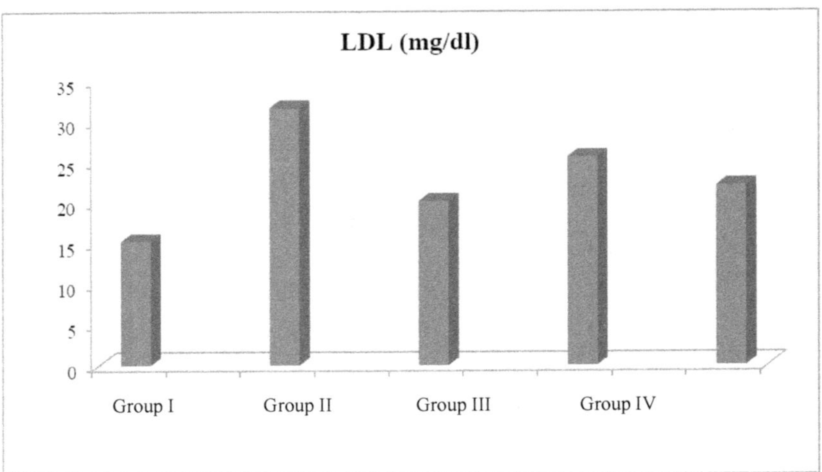


**Fig 42** Results of LDL Variation

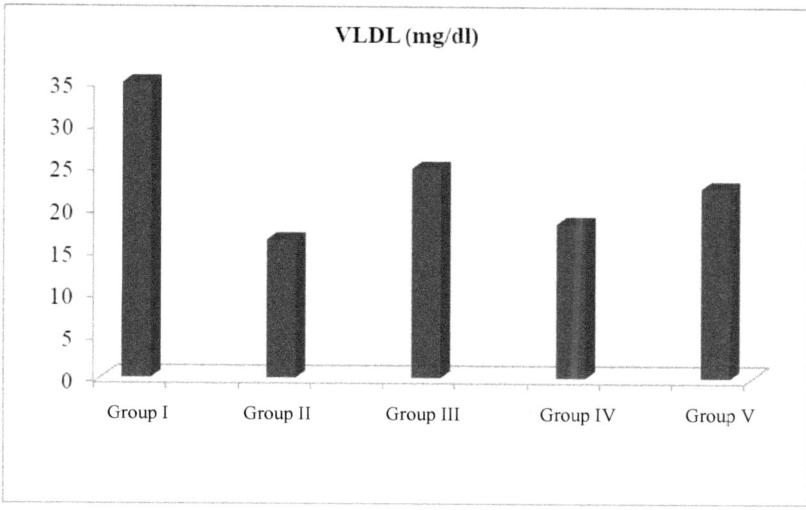


**Fig 43** Result of VLDL Variation

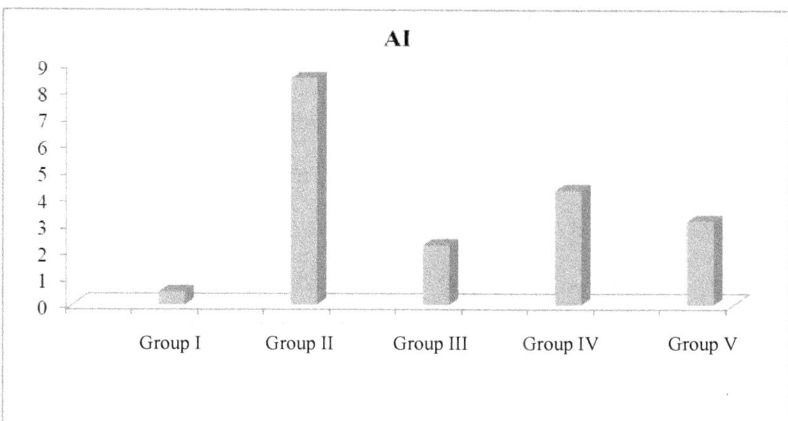


**Fig 44** AI Variation

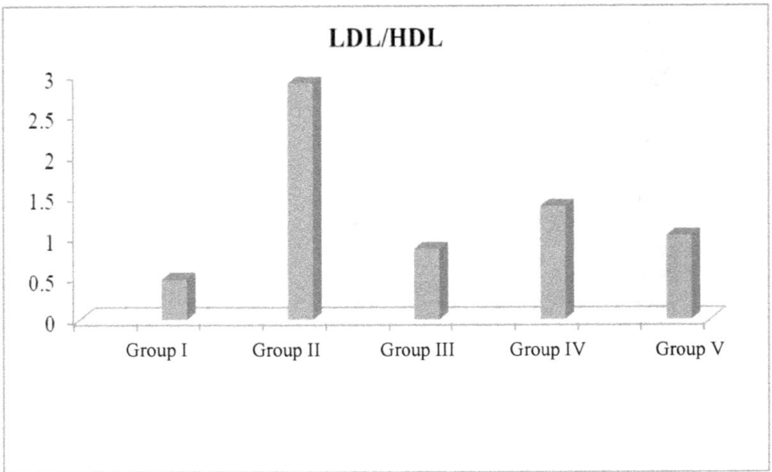


**Fig 45** Results of LDL / HDL Variation

The reduction of plasma total cholesterol is associated with decrease in its LDL fraction which is a major potentially modifiable risk factor of cardio vascular disease and the target of drug. Many suggest that the cholesterol lowering activity of this product appears to be due to the enhancement of LDL – C catabolism through hepatic receptors (Chidambaram and Kumarappan, 2007). In addition to herbal siddha formulation of Karuveppilai chooranam showed protective action which is reported to have a preventive function against atherosclerogenesis since an independent inverse relationship between blood HDL – C levels and cardio vascular risk incidence is reported (Khanna and Rizvi 2002). The lipoprotein called "good cholesterol" facilitates the mobilization of triglycerides and cholesterol from plasma to liver where it is catabolised and eliminated in the form of bile acids. The possible mechanism of this activity may result from the enhancement of Lecithin cholesteryl acyl transferase (LCAT) and inhibition of Hepatic Triglyceride Lipase (HTL) on HDL which may lead to a rapid catabolism of blood lipids through enterohepatic tissues (Anila and Vijayalakshmi 2002 ; Pritchard and Karpen 1986).

It is also recently reported that triglycerides plays a key role in the regulation of lipoprotein interaction to maintain normal lipid metabolism. Indeed, the elevated plasma TG levels were associated with an increased incidence of coronary artery disease Moreover these higher plasma TG levels have been attributed mainly to increase population of small, dense LDL deposits which are very atherogenic and enhanced cholesteryl ester mass transfer from apolipoprotein B containing lipoproteins (Austin *et al.*, 2017 ; Matafome and Loura 2011) TG has also been proposed to be major determinant of cholesteryl esterification, its transfer and HDL remodeling in human plasma (Guerin, 2001).

Herbal siddha formulation of KVC significantly suppresses the elevated blood concentration of TGs. This result suggests that the product is able to restore, at least partially, the catabolism of TG. The underlying the mechanism of this activity is not elucidated by the present study. However, as hypothesized by many works with other plants, the restoration of catabolic mechanism of TGs would be due to an increased stimulation of the lipolytic activity of Plasma Lipoprotein Lipase (Murakai and Longhli 1995).

Administration of herbal siddha formulation of Karuveppilai chooranamprovides a beneficial action on rat lipid metabolism with regard to the reduction of AI. Infact, the AI was decreased in all treated groups. Similar results were reported by others when studying the hypolipidemic effects of natural products (Perez *et al.*, 1999). This ameliorative action was due to the plasma lipid lowering activity of different constituents of the plant.

It is also desirable to have higher plasma HDL and lower LDL – C to prevent atherogenesis, since there is a positive correlation between an increased LDL – C / HDL – C ratio and the development of atherosclerosis. Again, the administration of herbal siddha formulation of Karuveppilai chooranam significantly suppress the higher values of LDL – C

/ HDL – C ratio showing the beneficial effect of this plant in preventing atherosclerosis incidence.

This result is considered as important for the treatment of hyperlipidemia induced atherosclerosis and apparently validates the folk medicinal use of hyperlipidemic patients in India.

## 5.4 Antidiabetic Activity Studies.

### 5.4 (a) Results of *in vitro* antihyperglycemic activity of KVC

The control showed glucose uptake at 0.9%, while for Rosiglitazone the glucose uptake was found to be 121.58% and for KVC with 100 and 200 µg/ml concentrations resulted in glucose uptake of 33.44% and 64.46% respectively (Table 26; Fig 46).

**Table 26** *In-vitro* glucose uptake studies for KVC using L-6 cell line

| S. No | Name Of The Test Substances | Test Conc.In µg/Ml | Protein Content | Glucose Uptake Percentage (%) | | |
|---|---|---|---|---|---|---|
| | | | | N1 | N2 | Averege |
| 1. | Control | - | 959.84 | 1.79±2.2 | 0.01±0.77 | 0.9 |
| 2. | Stg (Rosiglutozone) | 100 | 987.93 | 118.15±3.46 | 125.02±3.08 | 121.58 |
| 3. | KVC | 200 | 987.93 | 64.19±3.53 | 64.74±3.68 | 64.46 |
| | | 100 | 940.87 | 32.40±2.79 | 33.48±1.12 | 33.44 |

**Fig 46** Glucose uptake assay of KVC using L6 cell line

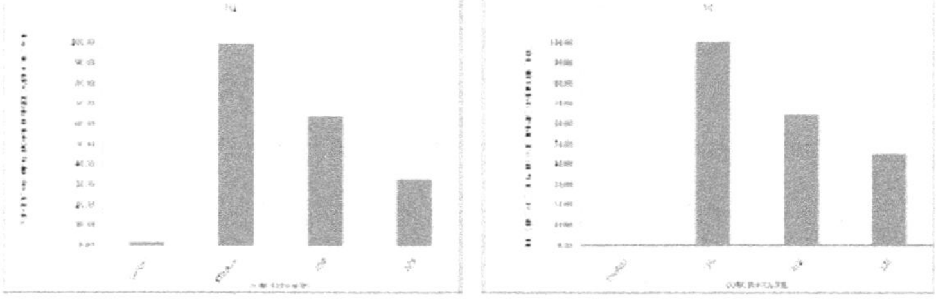

## *In Vivo* Antidiabetic Activity of KVC

Table 27, Fig 48 and Fig 49 illustrate the levels of initial and final blood glucose, and changes in body weight, in normal and treatment control animals in each group. The mean body weight of diabetic rats (G2) had significantly decreased as compared to normal control rats. The body weight of diabetic control rats treated with KVC at a dose of 100mg/kg and 200mg/kg had increased non-significantly as compared to normal control animals (Fig 47). Fasting blood glucose level had significantly increased to 214.46 ± 5.82 in diabetic animals as compared to normal animals (Table 27).

**Table 27** Effect Of KVC Initial And Final Body Weight and Blood Glucose In Normal And Treated Animals

| Group | Body Weight (G) | | Blood Glucose (Mg / 100ml) Initial | Blood Glucose (Mg / 100ml) |
|---|---|---|---|---|
| | Initial | Final | | Final |
| G1 | 235 ± 6.05 | 242 ± 6.10 | 86.60 ± 3.45 | 91.75 ± 3.18 |
| G2 | 225 ± 5.54 | 170 ± 7.25**(a) | 88.30 ± 3.70 | 214.46 ± 5.82**(a) |
| G3 | 232 ± 7.44 | 238 ± 7.30 | 90.64 ± 4.25 | 124.45 ± 4.35**(b) |
| G4 | 230 ± 7.20 | 240 ± 7.35 | 88.75 ± 3.65 | 146.45 ± 7.25**(b) |
| G5 | 230 ± 7.35 | 238 ± 7.35 | 90.42 ± 3.62 | 155.48 ± 4.62**(b) |

- Values are expressed as mean ± SEM.
- Values were compared by using analysis of variance (ANOVA) followed by Newman-Keul's multiple range tests.
- ** (a) Values are significantly different from normal control G1 at P<0.001.

** (b) Values are significantly different from Diabetic control G2 at P<0.01.

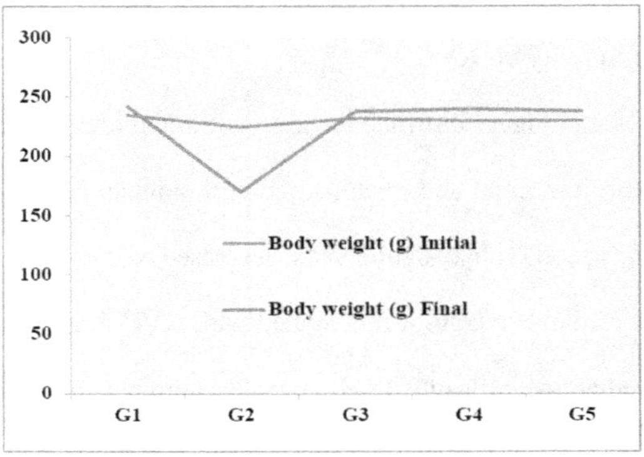


**Fig 47** Graphical Representatio Of BMI Variation

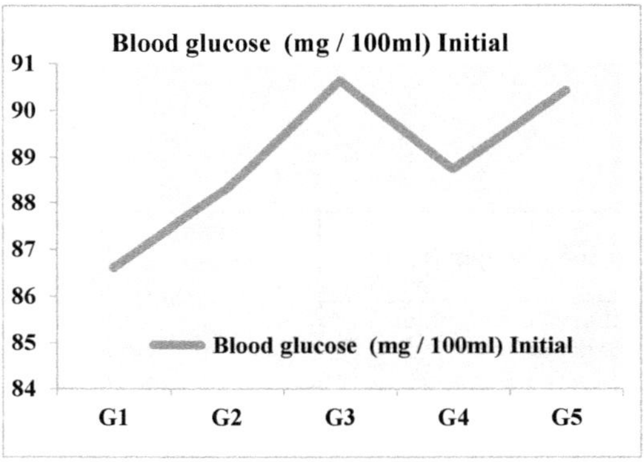


**Fig 48** Intial Blood Glugose Level Variation

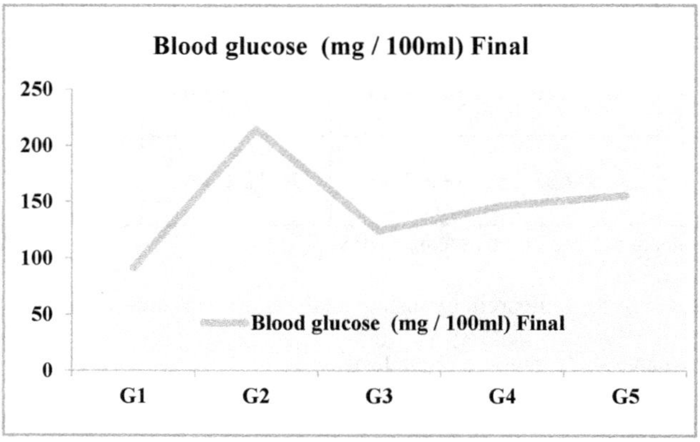


**Fig 49** Final Blood Glucose Variation

However, the level of fasting blood glucose, returned to near normal range in diabetic rats treated with KVC at a dose of 100mg/kg and 200mg.

Anti hyperglycemic activity of Kariveppillai choornam in STZ induced Diabetic Male albino wister rats(180-220gm). Each group IV and V treated with 100 to 200 mg/kg/bw KVC was used in 28 days. After 29th day found Haemoglobin,Glycosylated haemoglobin (HbA1c) and plasma level had decreased in Group IV and GroupV when compared to Group I,II and III. (Ags 50-52). HbA1c% and Plasma insulin (μU/ml) level had decreased in diabetic model rat and the values of HbA1c and Plasma insulin were significantly reduced in 100 mg and 200mg of KVC, ie 12.54±0.92,0.50±0.08, 30.80±2.60 and 12.64±1.22, 0.45±0.04, 29.70±2.60 (Table 28).

**Table 28** Effect Of KVC On Plasma Insulin, Haemoglobin And Glycosylated Haemoglobin In Normal And Treated Animals

| Groups | Haemoglobin (Gm/100ml) | Glycosylated Haemoglobin Hba$_1$ (%) | Plasma Insulin (μu/ml) |
|---|---|---|---|
| G1 | 13.80 ± 1.52 | 0.40 ± 0.06 | 33.48 ± 2.75 |
| G2 | 6.65 ± 0.52**(a) | 0.90 ± 0.14**(a) | 13.58 ± 1.60**(a) |
| G3 | 14.30 ± 1.30**(b) | 0.42 ± 0.07**(b) | 32.35 ± 2.42**(b) |
| G4 | 12.54 ± 0.92**(b) | 0.50 ± 0.08**(b) | 30.80 ±2.60**(b) |
| G5 | 12.64 ± 1.22**(b) | 0.45 ± 0.04**(b) | 29.70 ± 2.60**(b) |

Values are expressed as mean ± SEM.Values were compared by using analysis of variance (ANOVA) followed by Newman-Keul's multiple range tests. ** (a) Values are significantly different from normal control G1 at P<0.001. ** (b) Values are significantly different from Diabetic control G2 at P<0.01.

**Fig 50** Haemoglobin Variation among 5 groups of test organisms after KVC treatment

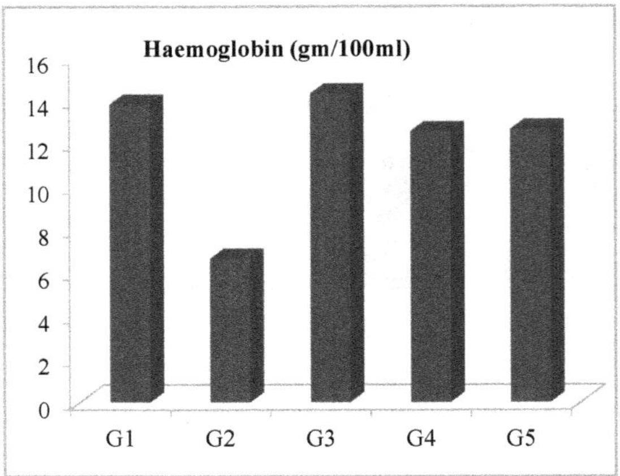


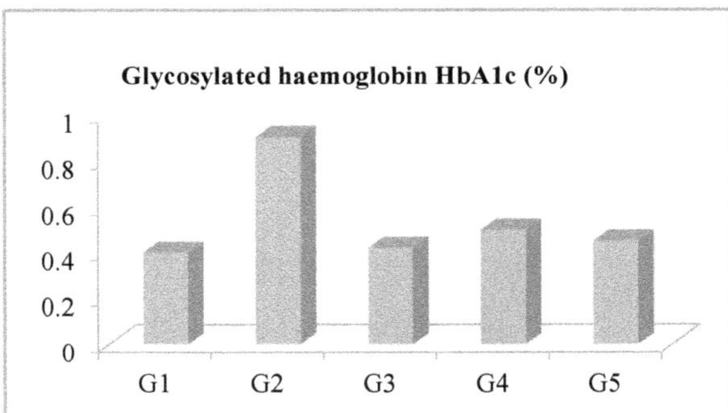


**Fig 51** HbA1c Variation among 5 groups of test organisms after KVC treatment.

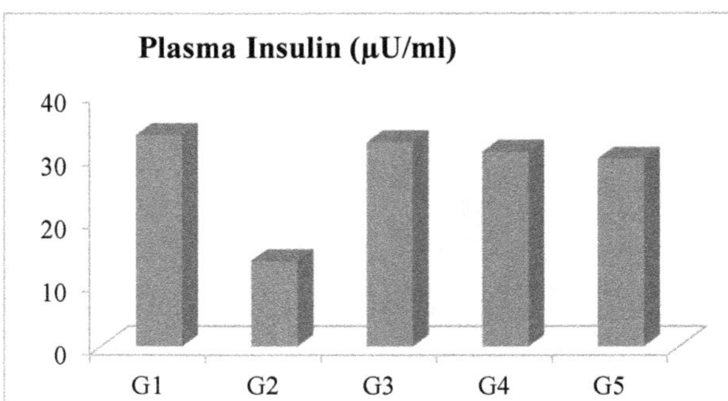


**Fig 52** Plasma Insulin Variation among 5 groups of test organisms after KVC treatment.

Table 28 illustrates the levels of total hemoglobin, glycosylated hemoglobin and plasma insulin in normal rat and treatment control animals in each group.

The levels of total hemoglobin, and plasma insulin levels decreased significantly where as glycosylated heamoglobin levels increased significantly as compared to normal control rats. However, the level of total hemoglobin, glycosylated hemoglobin and plasma insulin, returned to near normal range in diabetic rats treated with KVC at a dose of 100mg/kg and 200mg/kg.

The level of serum total cholesterol (TC), triglycerides (TG), high density lipoprotein (HDL), Low density lipoprotein (LDL) and phospholipids of normal and experimental animals in each group.Total cholesterol, triglycerides, high density lipoprotein, Low density lipoprotein (LDL) and phospholipids levels were significantly increased in Group II & III, where as HDL-C level was decreased in streptozotocin induced diabetic rats (Group II) as compared to normal rats. Treatment of normal and streptozotocin induced diabetic rats with KVC at a dose of 100mg/kg and 200mg/kg for 28 days resulted in marked decrease in total cholesterol, triglycerides, Low density lipoprotein (LDL) and phospholipids levels and increase in HDL-C levels as compared to streptozotocin induced diabetic rats.ie from 228.48±7.52, 160.65 ±4.65, 35.60±1.34, 220.48±6.30, 42.65±2.50 (GIII) to 123.40±3.35, 104.65±2.80, 40.25±1.58, 153.40±3.82 and 28.35±1.76 (Group V) respectively.

**Table 29** Serum Lipids Of Normal And Experimental Groups of organisms after KVC

| GROUPS | Total Cholesterol (mg/dl) | Triglyceride (mg/dl) | HDL-C (mg/dl) | Phospholipids (mg/dl) | LDL (mg/dl) |
|---|---|---|---|---|---|
| **G1** | 88.80 ± 2.68 | 92.48 ± 2.65 | 56.50 ± 1.85 | 125.65 ± 2.43 | 18.35 ± 1.40 |
| **G2** | 228.48 ± 7.52**(a) | 160.65 ± 4.65**(a) | 35.60 ± 1.34**(a) | 220.48 ± 6.30**(a) | 42.65 ± 2.50**(a) |
| **G3** | 118.90 ± 3.36**(b) | 98.90 ± 2.46**(b) | 45.20 ± 1.45 | 154.45 ± 3.95 | 27.80 ± 1.80**(b) |
| **G4** | 130.60 ± 3.58**(b) | 120.86 ± 2.90**(b) | 43.25 ± 1.38**(b) | 162.60 ± 4.15**(b) | 33.28 ± 1.55**(b) |
| **G5** | 123.40 ± 3.35**(b) | 104.65 ± 2.80**(b) | 40.25 ± 1.58**(b) | 153.40 ± 3.82**(b) | 28.35 ± 1.76**(b) |

- Values are expressed as mean ± SEM.
- Values were compared by using analysis of variance (ANOVA) followed by Newman-Keul's multiple range tests.
- ** (a) Values are significantly different from normal control G1 at P<0.001.

  ** (b) Values are significantly different from Diabetic control G2 at P<0.01.

## Results Of *In vivo* Antidiabetic Activity Studies Of Test Organisms

### Effect of Karivepillai Chooranam on Glycogen Content

Glycogen content of liver tissue was estimatted on the 28$^{th}$day in non diabetic control, diabetic controle drug, treated group, and possitive controle group as shown in table 3.91f.

**Table 30** Effect Of Karuveppillai Chooranam On Glycogen Content (mg/gm tissue) of 5 groups of test organisms

| S.No | Groups | Liver Tissue Glycogen Content (mg/g tissue) |
|---|---|---|
| 1 | Group I | $44.30 \pm 3.50$ |
| 2 | Group II | $12.28 \pm 0.82^{*\varepsilon}$ |
| 3 | Group III | $36.50 \pm 1.74^{*ɔ}$ |
| 4 | Group IV | $28.40 \pm 1.35^{*b}$ |
| 5 | Group V | $30.59 \pm 1.50^{*b}$ |

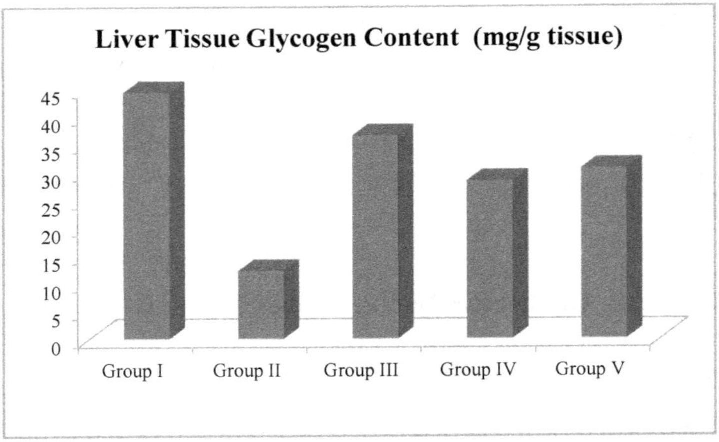


**Fig 53** Results Of Liver Tissue Glycogen Content Of 5 Groups Of Test Organisms

- Values are expressed as mean ± SEM.
- Values were compared by using analysis of variance (ANOVA) followed by Newman-Keul's multiple range tests.
- ** (a) Values are significantly different from normal control G1 at $P<0.001$.

  ** (b) Values are significantly different from Diabetic control G2 at $P<0.01$.

In the diabetic control, rats liver glycogen content decreased significantly by 79.89 % as compared to non-diabetic control. Treatment with Glipizide, KVC at a dose of 100mg/kg and 200mg/kg led to 74.47 %, 66.05 % and 68.79% increase in liver glycogen content in comparison to diabetic control, i.e., Group III Liver tissue Glycogen content is 36.50±1.74 mg/g tissue led to 28.40±1.35 and 30.59±1.50 mg/g tissue (Group IV,V) respectively. (Table 30)

**Effect of KVC on Hepatic Enzymes**

The plasma glucose was determined 72hr after alloxan administration. Only those rats with over 180 mg% were included in the study. On the 28th day, hepatic enzymes Hexokinase, Glucokinase and substrate Glucose-6-phosphate were estimated in saline control (group I), diabetic control (group II) and treatment controls (groups III, IV and V).

The results were been compiled and presented in Table 31. As compared to non-diabetic control values, mean level of enzymes Hexokinase, Glucokinase and substrate Glucose-6-phosphate values decreased in diabetic control. The respective percentage decrease was 56.19%, 79.96% and 67.69% in diabetic control. Treatment with KVC at a dose of 100mg/kg and 200mg/kg for 28 days led to rise in percentage of these parameter by 22.03%, 56.03%, and 45.21% , 47.5%, 33.33% and 67.88% respectively (P<0.001) as compared to diabetic control. Also, treatment with Glipizide 10mg/kg for 28 days led to rise in percentage of these parameters by 27.55%, 65.39% and 58.0% respectively (P< 0.001) as compared to diabetic control.

**Table 31** Effect Of Karuveppillai Chooranam On Enzymes Involved In Carbohydrate Metabloism In Rats

| S.No | Groups | Hexokinase (µg/mg) | Glucose-6-Phosphate (µg/mg) | Glucokinase (µg/mg) |
|---|---|---|---|---|
| 1 | **Group I** | 0.215 ± 0.014 | 0.395 ± 0.012 | 27.38± 1.40 |
| 2 | **Group II** | 0.093 ± 0.005*[a] | 0.130 ± 0.008*[a] | 6.62 ± 0.30*[a] |
| 3 | **Group III** | 0.131 ± 0.008*[b] | 0.306 ± 0.012*[b] | 19.22 ± 0.90*[b] |
| 4 | **Group IV** | 0.125 ± 0.006*[b] | 0.234 ± 0.006*[b] | 16.10 ± 0.45*[b] |
| 5 | **Group V** | 0.144 ± 0.007*[b] | 0.245 ± 0.007*[b] | 16.30 ± 0.52*[b] |

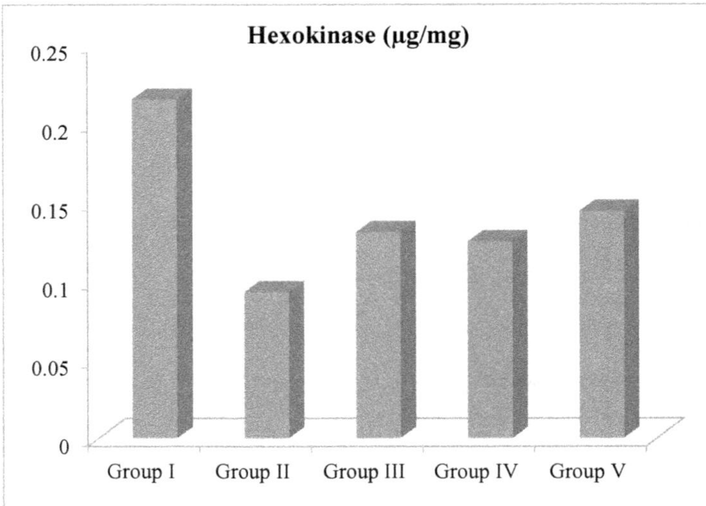


**Fig 54** Results of Hexokinase obtainted for the 5 groups of test organisms after KVC treatment

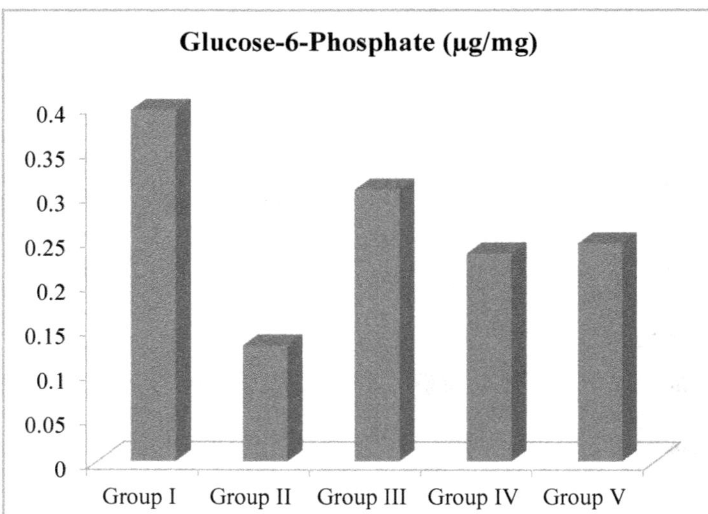


**Fig 55** Results of Glucose 6 Phosphate obtainted for the 5 groups of test organisms after KVC treatment

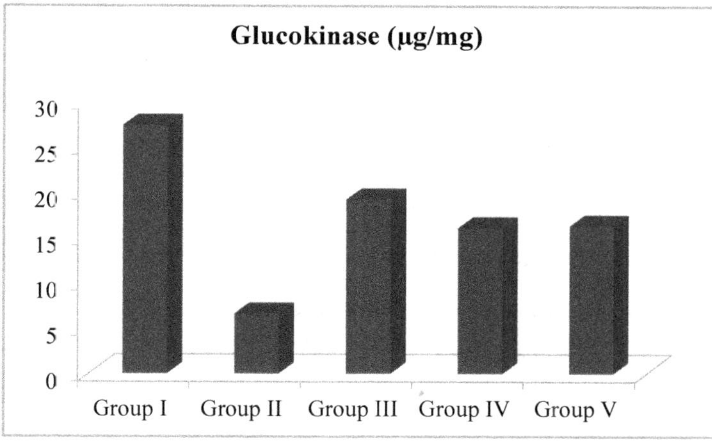


**Fig 56** Results of Glucokinase obtainted for the 5 groups of test organisms after KVC treatment

Values are expressed as mean ± SEM.

- Values were compared by using analysis of variance (ANOVA) followed by Newman-Keul's multiple range tests.
- ** (a) Values are significantly different from normal control G1 at P<0.001.
  ** (b) Values are significantly different from Diabetic control G2 at P<0.01.

## Effect Of Karuveppilai Chooranam Treatment On Biochemical Paramter In Streptozotocin Induced Rats

In liver homogenate, there was significant decrease in SOD, CAT and GPx levels and increase in LPO levels were observed in animals treated with streptozotocin 25mg/kg (group II) as compared to normal control group (Group I).Pre treatment with KVC at a dose of 100mg/kg and 200mg/kg orally for 28 days increase the levels of above indices like SOD,CAT and GPX levels and decrease levels of LPO significantly (P<0.01) in group III, IV and V (Table 32 and Figs 57-59). This suggests that KVC has effective antioxidative effects and could Scavenge well excess free radicals, which may prevent oxidative damage of the tissues and can increase a protective effect on improving diabetic complications (coronary atherosclerosis).

Hyperglycemia impairs the prooxidant/antioxidant levels (Argano and Brignardello, 1995). Free radicals react with lipids and cause peroxidative changes that result in enhanced lipid peroxidation (Girotti,1985).The antioxidant scavenging enzymes superoxidase dismutase (SOD),Catalase (CAT) and Glutathione peroxidase (GPX) offer protection to cells and tissues against oxidative injury (Bonnefont-Rousselot and Bostard, 2000).

**Table 32** Results of Antioxidant enzymes of the 5 groups of test organisms

| S.No | Group. No. | SOD (U/mg) Protein | CATALASE (U/mg) Protein | GPx (U/mg) Protein | LPO (U/mg) Protein |
|---|---|---|---|---|---|
| 1 | I | 135.30± 2.40 | 295.45± 2.40 | 1.22± 0.08 | 3.96± 0.18 |
| 2 | II | *a 73.26± 1.43 | *a 195.80± 2.75 | *a 0.45± 0.03 | *a 7.48± 0.15 |
| 3 | III | *b 123.10± 2.82 | *b 265.45± 1.90 | *b 0.91± 0.05 | *b 5.56± 0.15 |
| 4 | IV | *b 97.50± 1.65 | *b 235.10± 1.75 | *b 0.70± 0.04 | *b 5.65± 0.30 |
| 5 | V | *b 110.68± 2.65 | *b 245.80± 2.70 | *b 0.75± 0.05 | *b 4.90± 0.07 |

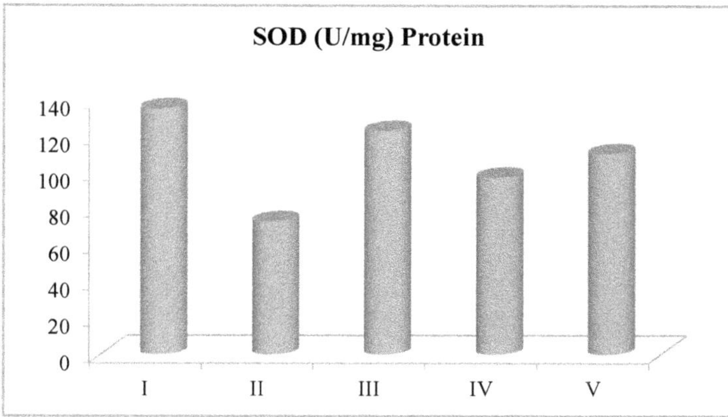


**Fig 57** Results of Super Oxidase Disumutase of the 5 groups of test organisms

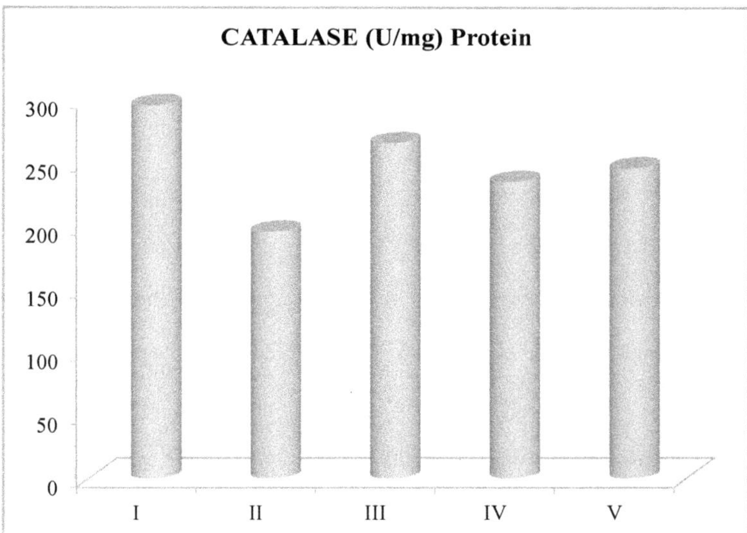


**Fig 58** Results of castalse protein of the 5 groups of test organisms

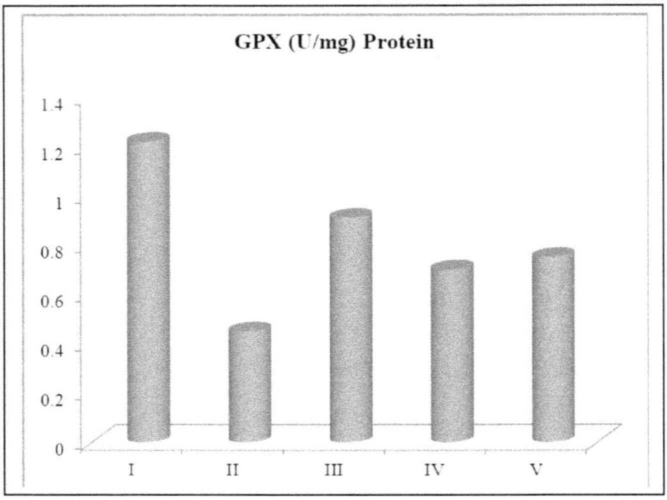


**Fig 59** Results of Glutathione Peroxide of the 5 groups of test organisms

Streptozotocin causes massive reduction in insulin release by of β-cells of the islets of Langerhans due to the destraction of β-cells. The mechanism of Streptozotocin action was fully described elsewhere (Lazarow, 1964). In our study, we have observed a significant increase in the plasma insulin level when Streptozotocin induced diabetic rats were treated with KVC at a dose of 100mg/kg and 200mg/kg. This could be due to potentiation of the insulin effect of plasma by increasing the pancreatic secretion of insulin from existing β- cells of islets of Langerhans or its release from bound insulin.

In uncontrolled or poorly controlled diabetes, there is an increased glycosylation of a number of proteins including haemoglobin and α-crystalline to aproximately 16% of lens (Alberti and Press, 1982). Glycosylated haemoglobin ($HbA_1C$) was found to increase in patients with diabetes mellitus to approximately 16% (Koenig and Peteson, 1976) and the amount of increase is directly proportional to the fasting blood glucose level (Jackson and

Hess, 1979). During diabetes the excess glucose present in blood reacts with haemoglobin. Therefore, the total haemoglobin level is decreased in Streptozotocin induced diabetic rats (Sheela and Augusti, 1992). Administration of KVC at a dose of 100mg/kg and 200mg/kg for 28 days prevents a significant elevation in glycosylated haemoglobin thereby increasing the level of total haemoglobin in diabetic rats. This could be due to the result of improved glycaemic control produced by KVC at a dose of 100mg/kg and 200mg/kg.

The body weight decreases in Streptozotocin diabetic rats. KVC at a dose of 100mg/kg and 200mg/kg increases the body weight in Streptozotocin induced diabetic rats. The ability of KVC at a dose of 100mg/kg and 200mg/kg to protect massive body weight loss seems to be due to its ability to reduce hyperglycemia.

The level of serum lipids are usually elevated in diabetes mellitus, and such an elevation represents the risk of coronary heart disease (CHD). Lowering of serum lipids concentration through diet or drug therapy seems to be associated with a decrease in the risk of vascular disease.The abnormal high concentration of serum lipids in diabetic subject is mainly due to the increased mobilization of free fatty acids from the peripheral fat depots, since insulin inhibits the hormone sensitive lipase. However, glucagon, catecholamines and other hormones enhance lipolysis. The marked hyperlipidaemia that characterized the diabetic state may therefore be regarded as a consequence of the uninhibited actions of lipolytic hormones on the fat deposits.

In the Streptozotocin -induced diabetes mellitus, the rise in blood glucose is accompanied by an increase in serum cholesterol and triglycerides. The levels of cholesterol and triglycerides and Low density lipoprotein (LDL) levels were brought to near normal by the treatment with KVC at a dose of 100mg/kg and 200mg/kg in Streptozotocin induced diabetic rats.

The effect of **Karuveppilai chooranam** at a dose of 100mg/kg and 200mg/kg on diabetic hypertriglyceridemia could be through its control of hyperglycaemia. This is in agreement with the facts that:

1. The level of glycaemic control is the major determinant of total and very low density lipoprotein (VLDL), and triglyceride, concentrations (Laakso, 1995).
2. Improved glycemic control following sulfonyl urea therapy decreases the levels of serum VLDL and total triglycerides (Taskinen, 2002; Taskinen and Beltz, 1986)

The main 'anti-atherogenic' lipoprotein (HDL) is involved in the transport of cholesterol from peripheral tissues into liver (Segal and Pachorick, 1984) and thereby it acts as a protective factor against coronary heart disease (Gordon and Castelli, 1977; Anila and Vijayalakshmi, 2002).

The level of HDL-cholesterol had decreased in diabetic rats when compared with normal rats (Pushparaj and Tan, 2000). Our results clearly showed that the level of HDL-cholesterol increased in Streptozotocin induced diabetic rats when treated with KVC a dose of 100mg/kg and 200mg/kg. These results suggest that KVC at a dose of 100mg/kg and 200mg/kg has protective effect against Streptozotocin induced diabetes and its complications.

As reported earlier (Welihinda and Karunanayake, 1986) in the current study also the liver glycogen content reduced significantly in diabetic control as compared to non-diabetic control. Treatment wit KVC at a dose of 100mg/kg and 200mg/kg prevented this alteration in glycogen content of liver tissue, but could not normalize the content of glycogen of the non-diabetic control. This prevention or depletion of glycogen in liver is possibly due to either stimulation of insulin release from β-cells (Lolitkar and Rao, 1966) or due to the insulinomimetic activity of some components of the plants resulting in direct peripheral glucose uptake.

Decreased enzymatic activity of Hexokinase, Glucokinase and substrate glucose-6-phosphate has been reported in diabetic animals resulting in the depletion of liver and muscle glycogen (Hikino and Kobayashi, 1989). The present study also had similar results. Treatment with KVC at a dose of 100mg/kg and 200mg/kg significantly increased the Hexokinase, Glucokinase activity and Glucose-6-phosphate level in the liver, indicating an overall increase in glucose influx thus KVC at a dose of 100mg/kg and 200mg/kg seems to have an overall effect of increase in glucose utilization.

Oxidative stress is an imbalance between reactive oxygen species and the antioxidant defense mechanisms of a cell or tissue, which leads to lipid peroxidation, DNA damage, and the inactivation of many enzymes (Speaker and Fabris, 1997). The enzymatic antioxidant defense system is the natural protector against lipid peroxidation that includes superoxide dismutase, catalase and glutathione peroxidase. Reduced activities of these enzymes in the tissue of streptozotocin toxic rats were observed in our study. Superoxide dismutase protects against the superoxide radical (O2·−), which damages the membrane and its biological structure. Catalase primarily decomposes hydrogen peroxide to $H_2O$ at a much faster rate, sharing this function with glutathione peroxidase. Glutathione peroxidase may play an important role in the removal of lipid hydroperoxides (Blokhina and Virolainen, 2003; Larson, 1988; Gutteridge, 1995) The balance between these enzymes is important for the efficient removal of oxygen radicals from tissues (Kokate *et al.*, 1990). Therefore, reduction in the activity of these enzymes may result in a number of deleterious effects due to the accumulation of superoxide radicals and $H_2O_2$. Significant increases in the activities of these enzymes were observed on KVC at a dose of 100mg/kg and 200mg/kg administration.

## 5.5 Cytotoxicity and Heavey Metal Studies

### *In-Vitro* Cytotoxic Study On Rat Skeletal Muscle L6 Cells

### Cytotoxic activity of KVC against L6 cell line

An *in vitro* cytotoxicity activity of Kariveppilai chooranam by glucose uptake assay Glucose uptake activity of test substance was determined in differentiated L6 cell line 80% confluence was observed in 40mm petri plates which were allowed to differentiate by maintaining in DMEM with 2% FBS for 4-6 days. The extent of differentiation was established by nucleation of cells. The differentiated cells were serum starved over night and at the time of experiment. The cells were washed with HEPES buffered Krebs Ringer Phosphate solution (KRP buffer) once and incubated with KRP buffer with 0.1% BSA for 30min at 37% toxic concentrations of test and standard drugs for 30 min along with control. 20μl of D-glucose solution was added simultaneously to each well and C for 30 min. After incubation, the uptake of the glucose was aspiration of solutions from wells and washed thrice with ice-cold KRP buffer solution. Cells with 0.1M NaOH solution and an aliquot of cell lysates were used to measure the cell associated glucose. The glucose levels in cell lysates were measured using glucose assay kit (ERBA). Two independent experimental HYvalues in duplicates were taken to determine the percentage enhancement of glucose uptake over controls.

**Table 33** The Cytotoxicity Values of KVC Against L6 Cell Line

| S.No | Test Conc. (μg/ml) | % Cytotoxicity | $CTC_{50}$(μg/ml) |
|---|---|---|---|
| 1 | 1000 | 62.62±1.0 | 448.01±5.0 |
| 2 | 500 | 57.46±1.3 | |
| 3 | 250 | 21.79±1.7 | |
| 4 | 125 | 15.79±0.6 | |
| 5 | 62.5 | 12.58±1.1 | |

GRAPHICAL REPRESENTATION

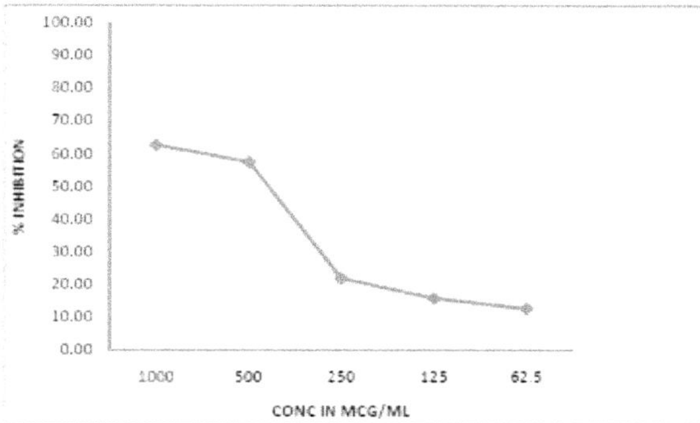


**Fig 60** Percentage Inhibition (%) of L6 Cell Line By KVC

As per Table 45, the increase in the test concentration resulted in graded cytotoxicity in the L6 cell line.Test concentration (μg/ml) of KVC from 62.5, to 125, 250, 500, and 1000 μg/ml produced cytotoxicity with gradual increase from .ie 12 58±1.1 to 15.79±0.6,21.79±1.7,57.46±1.3 and 62.62±1.0 respectivly. The CTC 50 was found to be 448.01 ± 5.0 μg/ml.

**Fig 61** Cytotoxicity Activity of KVC On L-6 Cell line

***In vitro*** **Cytotoxic Actvity Study On Mouse Embryo Plast Cells 3t3-L1 Cell Line Study**

**Table 34** The Cytotoxic Properties of KVC Against 3T3-L1 Cell Line

| S.No | Test conc (µg/ml) | % cytotoxicity | $CTC_{50}$(µg/ml) |
|---|---|---|---|
| 1 | 1000 | 69.22±0.2 | ≥1000 |
| 2 | 500 | 61.20±1.1 | |
| 3 | 250 | 19.53±1.4 | |
| 4 | 125 | 15.75±1.2 | |
| 5 | 62.5 | 9.92±2.6 | |

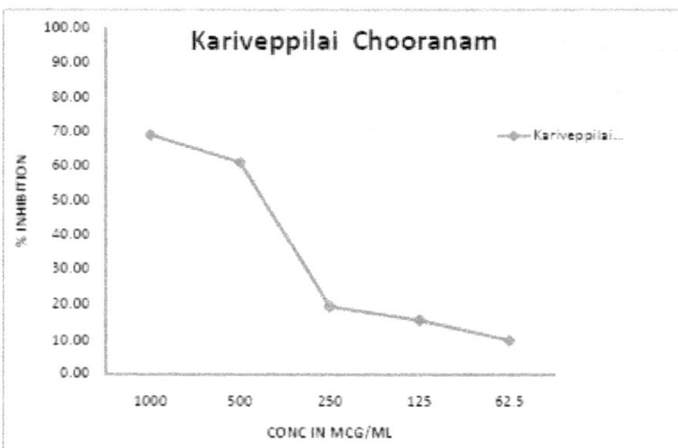


**Fig 62** Grapical Reprasentation of Cytotoxic Effect of Kariveppillai Chooranam (KVC) on 3T3 – L1 cell line

As per the Table 46, a gradual increase in the concentration resulted in graded cytotoxicity of 3T3-L1 cell line.The increasing the test concentration (µg/ml) of KVC, viz., 62.5,125,250,500, and 1000 µg/ml and showed cytotoxicity which increased gradually, ie, 9.92±2.6,15.75±1.2,19.53±1.4,61.20±1.1 and 69.22±0.2 respectively. CTC 50 was found to be >1000 µg/ml.

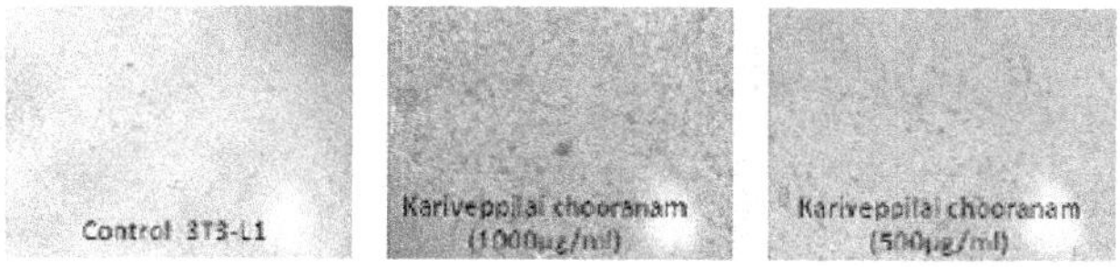


**Fig 63** Cytotoxic Activity of KVC

## HISTOPATHOLOGY

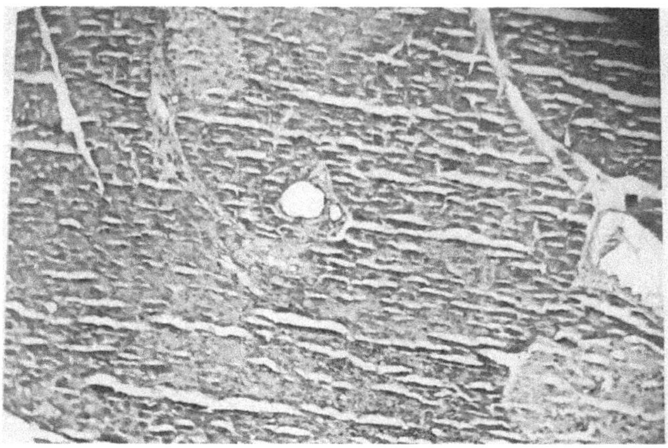

**Fig 64** Normal control rat (Normal Saline – 10ml)

The Normal numbers and volume of the islet cells

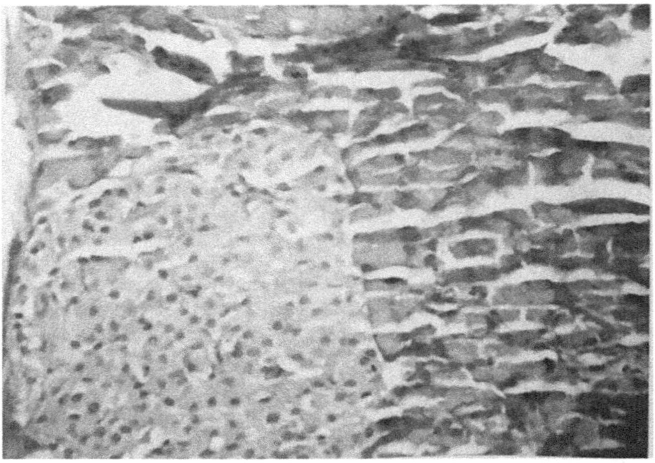

**Fig 65** Toxic control rat (Alloxan 150mg/kg)

The number of islet cells were severely decreased, islets cells were severly swelled

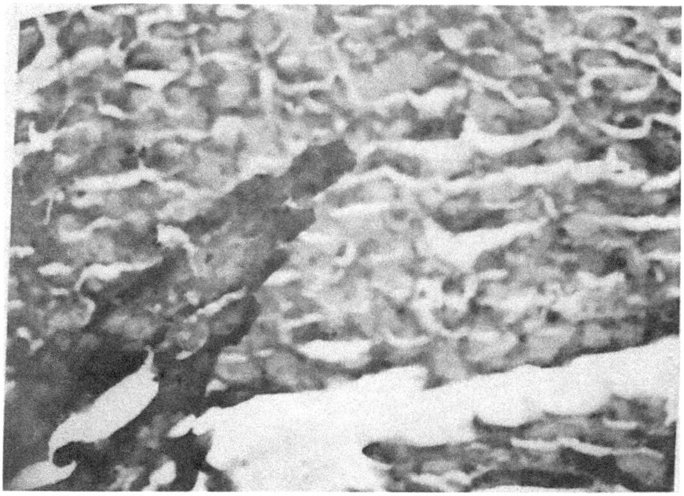

**Fig 66** Positive control (Glipizide 10 mg / Kg) Rat

The number of islet cells were mildly decreased, islets were mildly swelled

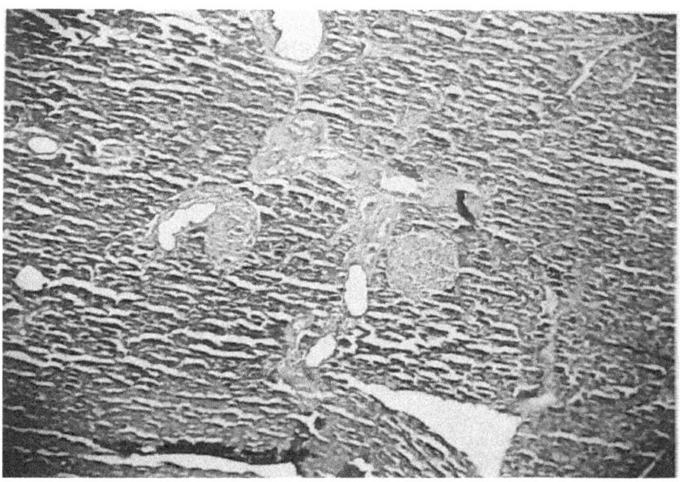

**Fig 67** Treatment Group (250mg/kg) Rat

The number of islet cells were moderately decreased, islet cells were moderately swelled

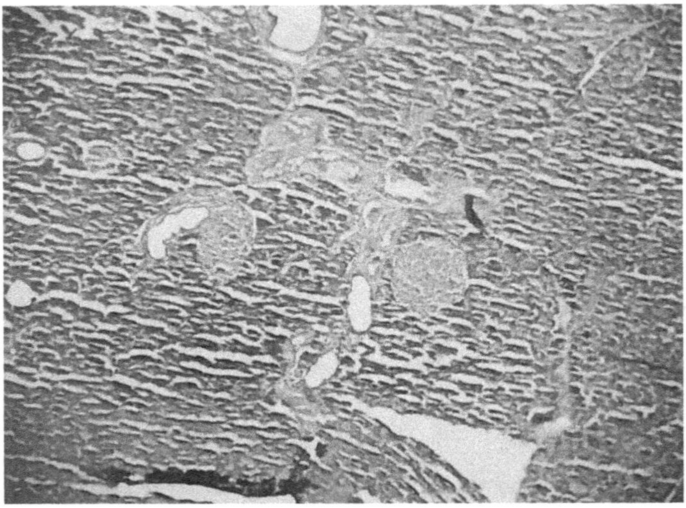

**Fig 68** Treatment Group (500mg/kg) Rat

The islet cells showing moderately decreased, swelled features.

## HEAVY METAL ANALYSIS

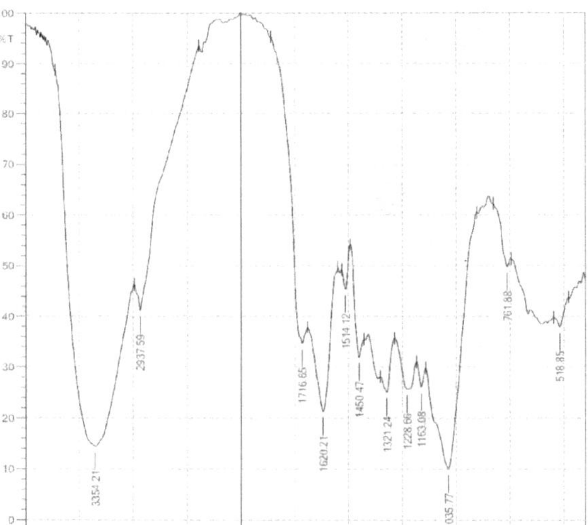


**Fig 69** FTIR Analysis graph of KVC

**Table 35** Correlation Between Wave Length and Chemical Bond

| Wave length | Bond | Chemical bond | Stretching(S) OR Bending(B) | Compound |
|---|---|---|---|---|
| 3354.21 | Medium | NH | S | Secondary amine |
| 2937.59 | Strong-broad | NH NH | S | Amine |
| 1716.65 | Strong | C-O | S | Carboxilic acid |
| 1620.21 | Strong | N-O | S | Nitro Compound |
| 1514.12 | Strong | N-O | S | Nitro Compound |
| 1450.42 | Medium | C-H | B | Alkane |
| 1321.24 | Medium | O-H | B | Phenol |
| 1228.66 | Strong | C-O | S | Vinyl ether |
| 1163.08 | Strong | C-O | S | Ester |
| 1035.77 | Strong | S=O | S | Sulfoxide |
| 761.88 | Strong | C-Br | S | Halo compound |
| 518.85 | Strong | C-1 | S | Halo compound |

FTIR results confirmed the presence of various bioactive molecules in KVC, The natural phytocompounds and secondary metabolites of Phenol (Harpreet Walia 2012, and Jasmit Kaur, Kathirvel and Sujatha 2012, Revathi and Jeyaseelan Senthilnath, 2014 ) amines, alkanes (Gopalakrishnan2011), carboxylic acid, aromatic rings (Jamwal and javed, 2013), nirto compounds, ester, and alkyl halides possess more therapeutic activities in Antioxidant, Antimicrobial, Anticancer and antiinflammatory properties respectively.

- **Phenol**: Phenolic groups act as an antioxidants. They inhibit free radicals and highly antimicrobial with antiseptic activities.
- **Amines:** Amines acts as neurotransmitters. They reduce the damaged cells and clear out necrotic cells. They are involved in protein synthesis.
- **Carboxylic Acid**: They exist in most living cells and help for some metabolic activities.

- **Alkenes:** Alkenes have little biological activity. They confer protection against bacteria and fungi.
- **Nitro compounds:** The Nitrile groups stimulated by the implication of aldosterone's role in several pathogenic diseases help regulate sodium pottasium balance, Extracellular fluid volume and Blood pressure.
- **Aromatics:** Aromatic hydrocarbons relieve the pain and reduce the inflammation.
- **Ester:** Esters are organic compounds formed when carboxylic acids combine with an alcohol and release water. Ester of Sitostanol decreases in cholesterol absorption.
- **Alkyl halides:** Alkyl halides are also known as haloalkanes. They required for the synthesis of glutathione and anti-oxidant activity.

**Table 36** Analysis of Functional Groups and its Absorbance

| Functional group | Wave length | Absorbance % |
|---|---|---|
| Aromatic C-H Bending(S) | 518.85 | 45.298271 |
| | 761.88 | 52.317328 |
| | 1035.77 | 29.136347 |
| | 1163.08 | 38.537465 |
| | 1228.66 | 38.327708 |
| | 1321.24 | 38.010405 |
| Aromatic C=C Bending(M.M) | 1450.47 | 42.180055 |
| | 1514.12 | 49.973853 |
| | 1620.21 | 35.786222 |
| | 1716.65 | 43.108960 |
| Alkyl-CH Stretch(M or S) | 2937.59 | 47.307174 |
| Alcohol,Phenol-OH Stretch (Broad S) | 3354.21 | 31.742696 |

**ICP – OES**

ICP-OES is a convenient technique to check the availability of essential trace elements in medicinal plants. The intensity of this emission is indicative of the concentration of the elements within the drug KVC.

**Table 37** Heavy Metal Analysis of KVC

| Elements Symbol | Wave Length(Nm) | Concentration(Mg/L) |
|---|---|---|
| Al | 396.152 | BDL |
| As | 188.979 | BDL |
| Ca | 315.807 | 82.150 |
| Cd | 228.802 | BDL |
| Cu | 327.393 | BDL |
| Fe | 238.204 | 05.016 |
| Hg | 253.652 | BDL |
| K | 766.491 | 33.024 |
| Mg | 285.213 | 01.244 |
| Na | 589.592 | 71.120 |
| Ni | 231.604 | BDL |
| Pb | 220.353 | BDL |
| P | 213.617 | 476.351 |
| S | 180.731 | 01.317 |
| Zn | 206.200 | 01.058 |

**The specification of Siddha, Ayurveda and Unani products intended for exports are summerized below:**

**BDL- Below Detecting Limit:**

1% = 10000 ppm, (1 ppm = 1/1000000 (or) 1 ppm = 0.0001%)

**The toxic metals and the permissible limits:**

| Heavy metals | WHO & FDA limits |
|---|---|
| ◉ Arsenic (As) | 10ppm |
| ◉ Mercury (Hg) | 1ppm |
| ◉ Lead (Pb) | 10ppm |
| ◉ Cadmium (Cd) | 0.3ppm |

❖ ICP-OES results of KVC show that the heavy toxic metals like Al, As, Cd, Cu, Hg, Ni, and Pb were detected and their concentrations were found to be present within the limits recommended by WHO, Genva, (2005). The minerals like calcium, iron, potassium, magnesium, sodium, phosphorus, sulphur and zinc are present (Nielson, 1987). The Cu, Mg, Se and Zn, polyphenols and Flavonoids play a significant role in curing human diseases (Schroeter and Boyd 2002). The Cu and Zn participated in the SOD mechanism that plays an important role in oxidative defence systems (Guo and Chen, 2011). A clinical study proved that Zn supplementation was more effective against Hepatitis C virus and acted as good antioxidants (Murakami and Koyabu, 2007).

**SEM ANALYSIS**

The scanning electron microscope (SEM) analysis of KVC was recorded. The SEM analysis revealed that the particles of KVC during varied in size from 1 μm to 10 μm (Fig 70 and 71)

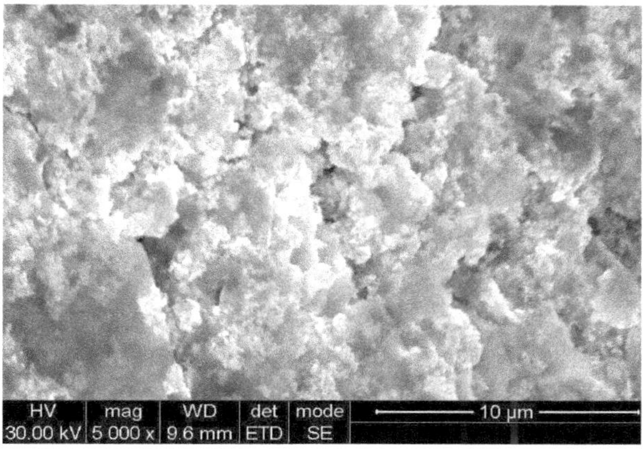


**Fig 70** SEM Analysis Showing particle size of 10 μm

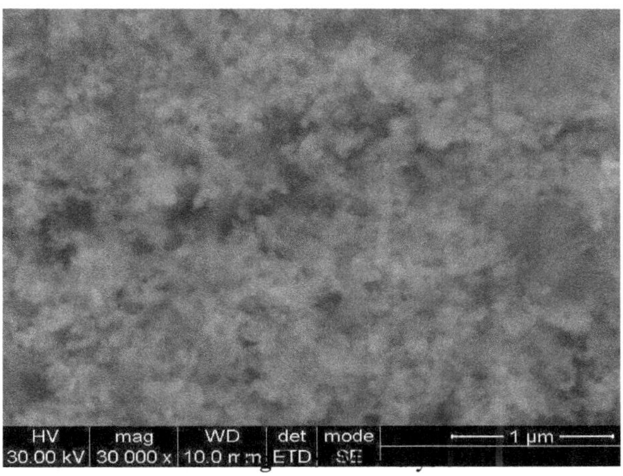


**Fig 71** SEM Analysis Showing particle size of 1 μm

The micro particles exhibit the following qualities:

- Sustained release of the drug during the transportation through absorption.
- Altering the distribution of the drug
- Subsequently clears the drug
- Increasing the drug therapeutic efficacy
- Increasing the bio-availability
- Reducing the side effects.

❖ So the minimal quantity of the medicine is enough to treat the diseased Hyperlipidemic state.

## 5.6 Clinical Trial Study

At the end of the open labeled single blind non randomized control study, the total cholesterol (TC), LDL, TGL and Randamized blood sugar levels were found decreased. There were no adverse side effects observed during the entire treatment period, *i. e.*, liver and renal parameters were within normal levels.

The statistical analysis for the clinical study is done for 17 cases including both inpatients and outpatients using the paired "t " test method.

**Table 38** The Results Of Blood Sugar Levels Of Two Groups Of The Clinical Study

| S. No | Value | Group 1 | Group 2 |
|---|---|---|---|
| 1. | MEAN | 259.2353 | 174.4906 |
| 2. | SD | 77.4827 | 54.9317 |
| 3. | SEM | 18.7923 | 13.3229 |
| 4. | N | 17 | 17 |

Group 1 – before treatment, Group 2- after treatment with the trial drug
SD – Standard Deviation, SEM – Standard error of mean, N – no of cases.

The statistical analysis for the blood sugar levels was done using the paired "t" test method and the results are given in Table 38. At 16 degrees of freedom the "t" value was 9.39, with a standard error of difference of 9.021. There exists a 95% of confidence interval.

The two tailed p value is less than 0.0001. The difference is considered to be extremely statistically significant. The trial drug has a significant difference in its antihyperglycemic action.

**Table 39** Results Of Total Cholesterol Levels.

| S. No | Value | Group 1 | Group 2 |
|---|---|---|---|
| 1. | MEAN | 218.741 | 187.547 |
| 2. | SD | 28.815 | 25.799 |
| 3. | SEM | 6.989 | 6.257 |
| 4. | N | 17 | 17 |

The statistical analysis of total cholesterol levels was done using the paired "t" test method and the results are given in Table 39. At 16 degrees of freedom the "t" value was 4.27, with a standard error of difference of 7.30. There exists a 95% of confidence interval. The two tailed p value equals 0.0006.The difference is considered to be extremely statistically significant. The trial drug has a significant difference in lowering the elevated total cholesterol levels.

**Table 40** Result Of HDL Cholesterol Levels.

| S. No | Value | Group 1 | Group 2 |
|---|---|---|---|
| 1. | MEAN | 38.941 | 38.800 |
| 2. | SD | 5.448 | 7.024 |
| 3. | SEM | 1.321 | 1.703 |
| 4. | N | 17 | 17 |

The statistical analysis for HDL cholesterol levels was done using the paired "t" test method and the results are given in Table 40. At 16 degrees of freedom the "t" value is 0.0615, with a standard error of difference of 2.29. The two tailed p value equals 0.95. The difference is not statistically significant.

**Table 41** Result Of LDL Cholesterol Levels.

| S. No | Value | Group 1 | Group 2 |
|---|---|---|---|
| 1. | MEAN | 126.512 | 108.565 |
| 2. | SD | 27.538 | 19.523 |
| 3. | SEM | 6.679 | 4.735 |
| 4. | N | 17 | 17 |

The statistical analysis of LDL cholesterol levels was don e using the paired "t" test method and the results are given in Table 41. At 16 degrees of freedom the "t" value was 1.95, with a standard error of difference of 9.21. The two tailed p value equals 0.069. The difference is not quite statistically significant.

**Table 42** Result Of VLDL Cholesterol Levels.

| S. No | Value | Group 1 | Group 2 |
|---|---|---|---|
| 1. | MEAN | 45.376 | 39.888 |
| 2. | SD | 20.637 | 17.876 |
| 3. | SEM | 5.005 | 4.336 |
| 4. | N | 17 | 17 |

The statistical analysis for VLDL cholesterol levels was done using the paired "t" test method and the results are given in Table 42. At 16 degrees of freedom the "t" value is 1.11, with a standard error of difference of 4.94. The two tailed p value equals 0.28. The difference is not statistically significant.

**Table 43** Result Of Triglyceride Levels.

| S. No | Value | Group 1 | Group 2 |
|---|---|---|---|
| 1. | MEAN | 230.865 | 190.029 |
| 2. | SD | 102.638 | 92.543 |
| 3. | SEM | 24.893 | 22.445 |
| 4. | N | 17 | 17 |

The statistical analysis for triglyceride cholesterol levels was done using the paired "t" test method and the results are given in Table 43. At 16 degrees of freedom the "t" value was 1.65, with a standard error of difference of 24.71. The two tailed p value equals 0.118. The difference is not statistically significant.

**Table 44** Result Of HbA1c Levels

| S. No | Value | Group 1 | Group 2 |
|---|---|---|---|
| 1. | MEAN | 9.600 | 7.782 |
| 2. | SD | 1.692 | 1.908 |
| 3. | SEM | 0.410 | 0.463 |
| 4. | N | 17 | 17 |

Group 1 – before treatment, Group 2- after treatment with the trial drug
SD – Standard deviation, SEM – Standard error of mean, N – no of cases.

The statistical analysis of the HbA1c levels was done using the paired "t" test method and the results are given in Table 44. At 16 degrees of freedom the "t" value was 9.65, with a standard error of difference of 0.19. There exists a 95% of confidence interval. The two tailed p value is less than 0.0001. The difference is considered to be extremely statistically significant.The trial drug has a significant difference in reducing elevated HbA1c levels.

The Pearson correlation between fasting blood sugar and post-prandial blood sugar showed significant effect of KVC at 0.01 level (2-tailed) (Table 45). Similarly, the Pearson correlation between HbA1c and lipids indicated the significance of KVC both at 0.01 level (2-tailed) and 0.05 level (2-tailed), indicating hypolipidemic activity of KVC (Table 46).

**Table 45** Changes In Blood Sugar At Fasting And Post-Prandial Levels Before And After

**Pearson Correlations**

| | | B.FBS | B.PPBS | B.SU | A.FBS | A.PPBS | A.SU |
|---|---|---|---|---|---|---|---|
| B.FBS | Pearson Correlation | 1 | .658** | -.057 | .906** | .831** | .005 |
| | Sig. (2-tailed) | | .002 | .813 | .000 | .000 | .984 |
| | N | 20 | 20 | 20 | 20 | 20 | 20 |
| B.PPBS | Pearson Correlation | .658** | 1 | -.091 | .698** | .774** | .013 |
| | Sig. (2-tailed) | .002 | | .704 | .001 | .000 | .957 |
| | N | 20 | 20 | 20 | 20 | 20 | 20 |
| B.SU | Pearson Correlation | -.057 | -.091 | 1 | -.052 | -.060 | .755** |
| | Sig. (2-tailed) | .813 | .704 | | .829 | .802 | .000 |
| | N | 20 | 20 | 20 | 20 | 20 | 20 |
| A.FBS | Pearson Correlation | .906** | .698** | -.052 | 1 | .893** | .113 |
| | Sig. (2-tailed) | .000 | .001 | .829 | | .000 | .636 |
| | N | 20 | 20 | 20 | 20 | 20 | 20 |
| A.PPBS | Pearson Correlation | .831** | .774** | -.060 | .893** | 1 | .159 |
| | Sig. (2-tailed) | .000 | .000 | .802 | .000 | | .503 |
| | N | 20 | 20 | 20 | 20 | 20 | 20 |
| A.SU | Pearson Correlation | .005 | .013 | .755** | .113 | .159 | 1 |
| | Sig. (2-tailed) | .984 | .957 | .000 | .636 | .503 | |
| | N | 20 | 20 | 20 | 20 | 20 | 20 |

**. Correlation is significant at the 0.01 level (2-tailed).

**Table 46** Pearson Correlation of $HbA_{1}c$ And Lipids

(**. Correlation is significant at 0.01 level (2-tailed) and * at 0.05 level (2-tailed)).

| Pearson Correlation | | | | | | | | | | | | | |
|---|---|---|---|---|---|---|---|---|---|---|---|---|---|
| | | B.HBA1C | B.TC | B.HDL | B.LDL | B.VLDL | B.TGL | A.HBA1C | A.TC | A.HDL | A.LDL | A.VLDL | A.TGL |
| B.HBA1C | Pearson Correlation | 1 | .089 | -.320 | .103 | .042 | .118 | .860** | .057 | -.233 | -.124 | -.031 | .264 |
| | Sig. (2-tailed) | | .709 | .169 | .665 | .859 | .621 | .000 | .812 | .322 | .603 | .896 | .261 |
| | N | 20 | 20 | 20 | 20 | 20 | 20 | 20 | 20 | 20 | 20 | 20 | 20 |
| B.TC | Pearson Correlation | .089 | 1 | .171 | .352 | .240 | .259 | .147 | .521* | -.111 | .678** | .181 | .274 |
| | Sig. (2-tailed) | .709 | | .470 | .127 | .308 | .270 | .535 | .019 | .643 | .001 | .446 | .243 |
| | N | 20 | 20 | 20 | 20 | 20 | 20 | 20 | 20 | 20 | 20 | 20 | 20 |
| B.HDL | Pearson Correlation | -.320 | .171 | 1 | .119 | -.378 | -.392 | -.139 | .028 | .140 | .018 | -.315 | -.102 |
| | Sig. (2-tailed) | .169 | .470 | | .617 | .100 | .087 | .560 | .907 | .557 | .939 | .176 | .668 |
| | N | 20 | 20 | 20 | 20 | 20 | 20 | 20 | 20 | 20 | 20 | 20 | 20 |
| B.LDL | Pearson Correlation | .103 | .352 | .119 | 1 | -.299 | -.289 | -.105 | .180 | -.355 | .229 | .067 | .233 |
| | Sig. (2-tailed) | .665 | .127 | .617 | | .200 | .216 | .660 | .449 | .125 | .331 | .778 | .323 |
| | N | 20 | 20 | 20 | 20 | 20 | 20 | 20 | 20 | 20 | 20 | 20 | 20 |
| B.VLDL | Pearson Correlation | .042 | .240 | -.378 | -.299 | 1 | .956** | .068 | .387 | .087 | .316 | .525* | .403 |
| | Sig. (2-tailed) | .859 | .308 | .100 | .200 | | .000 | .774 | .092 | 715 | .174 | .017 | .078 |
| | N | 20 | 20 | 20 | 20 | 20 | 20 | 20 | 20 | 20 | 20 | 20 | 20 |

| | | | | | | | | | | | | | |
|---|---|---|---|---|---|---|---|---|---|---|---|---|---|
| B.TGL | Pearson Correlation | .118 | .259 | -.392 | -.289 | .956** | 1 | .148 | .481* | .009 | .397 | .652** | .544* |
| | Sig. (2-tailed) | .621 | .270 | .087 | .216 | .000 | | .534 | .032 | .970 | .083 | .002 | .013 |
| | N | 20 | 20 | 20 | 20 | 20 | 20 | 20 | 20 | 20 | 20 | 20 | 20 |
| A.HBA1C | Pearson Correlation | .860** | .147 | -.139 | -.105 | .068 | .148 | 1 | .102 | -.179 | -.122 | .030 | .209 |
| | Sig. (2-tailed) | .000 | .535 | .560 | .660 | .774 | .534 | | .670 | .450 | .607 | .899 | .377 |
| | N | 20 | 20 | 20 | 20 | 20 | 20 | 20 | 20 | 20 | 20 | 20 | 20 |
| A.TC | Pearson Correlation | .057 | .521* | .028 | .180 | .387 | .481* | .102 | 1 | -.267 | .851** | .564** | .783** |
| | Sig. (2-tailed) | .812 | .019 | .907 | .449 | .092 | .032 | .670 | | .256 | .000 | .010 | .000 |
| | N | 20 | 20 | 20 | 20 | 20 | 20 | 20 | 20 | 20 | 20 | 20 | 20 |
| A.HDL | Pearson Correlation | -.233 | -.111 | .140 | -.355 | .087 | .009 | -.179 | -.267 | 1 | -.354 | -.240 | -.324 |
| | Sig. (2-tailed) | .322 | .643 | .557 | .125 | .715 | .970 | .450 | .256 | | .126 | .308 | .164 |
| | N | 20 | 20 | 20 | 20 | 20 | 20 | 20 | 20 | 20 | 20 | 20 | 20 |
| A.LDL | Pearson Correlation | -.124 | .678** | .018 | .229 | .316 | .397 | -.122 | .851** | -.354 | 1 | .414 | .531* |
| | Sig. (2-tailed) | .603 | .001 | .939 | .331 | .174 | .083 | .607 | .000 | .126 | | .069 | .016 |
| | N | 20 | 20 | 20 | 20 | 20 | 20 | 20 | 20 | 20 | 20 | 20 | 20 |
| A.VLDL | Pearson Correlation | -.031 | .181 | -.315 | .067 | .525* | .652** | .030 | .564** | -.240 | .414 | 1 | .750** |
| | Sig. (2-tailed) | .896 | .446 | .176 | .778 | .017 | .002 | .899 | .010 | .308 | .069 | | .000 |
| | N | 20 | 20 | 20 | 20 | 20 | 20 | 20 | 20 | 20 | 20 | 20 | 20 |
| A.TGL | Pearson Correlation | .264 | .274 | -.102 | .233 | .403 | .544* | .209 | .783** | -.324 | .531* | .750** | 1 |
| | Sig. (2-tailed) | .261 | .243 | .668 | .323 | .078 | .013 | .377 | .000 | .164 | .016 | .000 | |
| | N | 20 | 20 | 20 | 20 | 20 | 20 | 20 | 20 | 20 | 20 | 20 | 20 |

The 8 medicinal plants of KVC, according to Siddha principles have several qualities of panchabootha theory (Table 47). According to Siddha the hyperlipidemia condition is related to deranged "Thee" bhootham. The correction of the inequilibrium is made by substituting the drug which is predominantly of the opposite nature (ethirurai), a curative method employed by those drugs acting against the disease (Shanmugavelu, 1988). Most of the ingredients of KVC have predominant earth and air bhoothams.The predominant herbals of KVC possess earth and air which are responsible for normalizing the "Thee" (fire) bhootha in hyperlipidemia condition. Post absorptive taste (pirivu) of KVC is mainly the Pungent, and it prevents the excessive deposition of fat in the body.

**Table 47** Ingredients of Kariveppilai chooranam and Its Relation To Panchabhootham, Arusuvaikal and Thirithodam ( Incr - Increased; V – Vatham; P – Pitham; K – Kapham)

| Ingredients | Suvai | Thanmai | Pirivu | Panchabhootham | Thirithodam |
|---|---|---|---|---|---|
| Kariveppilai | Pungent | Hot | Pungent | Air+fire | Incr V<br>Incr P |
| Paruthivithai | Astringent<br>Sweet | Hot | Pungent | Earth+air<br>Earth+water | Incr V,P<br>Incr V |
| Manjal | Pungent<br>Bitter | Hot | Pungent | Air+fire<br>Air+space | Incr V,P<br>Incr V |
| Maramanjal | Bitter | Hot | Pungent | Air+space | Incr V |
| Kadukkai | Bitter<br>Pungent | Hot | Sweet | Air+space<br>Air+fire | Incr V<br>Incr P,V |
| Thantrikkai | Sour<br>Astringent | Cold | Sweet | Earth+fire<br>Earth+air | Incr P,<br>Incr V,K |
| Nellimulli | Sweet<br>Astringent<br>Sour | Cold | Sweet | Earth+water<br>Earth+air<br>Earth+fire | Incr K<br>Incr V,K<br>Incr P |
| Kadalazhinjil | Astringent | Cold | Pungent | Earth+air | Incr V,K |

# SUMMARY AND CONCLUSION

# 06 SUMMARY

The summay of major findings of the present research detailed in the thesis is given below:

Siddha medicinal plants refer to the herbals used in Siddha medicine to treat a wide range of human dieases. Several Siddha medicines are polyherbal preparations. Karivepillai Choornam (KVC) is prepared using 8 Siddha medicinal plants. KVC is clinically effective in diabetes and hyperlipidiamea.

Hence, the present research has concentrated on both *in vitro* and *in vivo* studies on the hypolipidemic and hypoglycemic propertices of KVC.

There are a number of studies on phytochemistry and pharmacology of 8 medicinal plants used in the Sastric preparation of KVC. The research literature available from 2000 onwards with reference to Siddha medicinal plants of KVC have been compiled.

Phytochemical and HPTLC fingerprint profile studies, antioxidant, antimicrobial, hypolipidemic and antidiabetic properties of KVC have been studied by using standard methods. The cytotoxicity and heavy metal analysis besides clinical trail of KVC were carried out.

The results of phytochemical studies on KVC revealed the presence of Alkaloids, Flavanoids, Saponins, Phenols, Steroids, Glycosides, Terpenoids and Tannins. While biochemical analysis showed the presence of Calcium, Sulphate, Chloride, Starch, Ferrous iron, Tannic acid, unsaturated compounds and Amino acid.

The HPTLC fingerprint profile studies displayed peaks corresponding to Rf values obtained for the different solvents extracts of KVC.

The results of ABTS, DBPH and Nitric oxide radical asssays of KVC had explained its antioxidant properties similar to those of reports of other antioxidant herbals studied by different researchers.

The antibacterial and antifungal potentials of KVC studied by agar well diffusion method have established the antimicrobial properties of KVC.

The antiadipogenesis studies and *in vivo* hypolipidemic activity of KVC compared with modern drug (atorvastatin) have proved the the effect of KVC in lowering cholesterol levels even at smaller dose (100 mg per kg body weight).

The *in vitro* anti hyperglycemic and *in vivo* antidiabetic studies have proved the statistically significant effect of KVC on hypolipidemia and diabetes.

The 3T3-L1 cell line studies showed the cytotoxicity of KVC exisiting within the permissible limits.

The FTIR studies for heavy metal analysis and ICP-OES technique for trace element analysis and SEM analysis for particle size of KVC have also proved that the KVC is a safe drug.

# 07. CONCLUSION

Karivepillai chooranam (KVC) is a polyherbal preparation of Siddha medicine. It is clinically proved to have hypolipidemic activity due to the properties of its Siddha herbals. The phytocompounds present in KVC have a combind effect in not only reducing the fat deposition (hypolipidemic) but also have (1) antioxidant, (2) antimicrobial and (3) antidiabetic properties. In addition, KVC does not possess heavy metals beyond the permissible limits.

According to Siddha principles, the KVC herbals dominate with the property of normalyzing hyperlipidemia and so it prevents the excessive deposition of fat in the body. Further investigations on the synergistic effect of the phytocompounds of the herbals in a Siddha drug like KVC will help in the discovery of new drug formulations to combat dreadful human diseases.

CPSIA information can be obtained
at www.ICGtesting.com
Printed in the USA
LVHW020012280423
745413LV00009B/210